A NEW BMI

Why Body Mind Intelligence Matters More than Body Mass Index

Peggy Norwood Stella, M.A.

First Edition September 2015

ISBN: 978-0692528358

The author/publisher has made every effort to acknowledge the research and body of knowledge that contributed to the ideas set forth in *A New BMI – Why Body Mind Intelligence Matters More than Body Mass Index*. Should this be proven impossible, then copyright holders are asked to contact the publisher so that suitable acknowledgment can be made at the first opportunity.

Disclaimer: *A New BMI – Why Body Mind Intelligence Matters More than Body Mass Index* provides guidance and a framework for health enhancement through physical activity and mindfulness practices. The guidance and advice contained within is to provide insight and not as a substitute for recommendations or treatments from your supervising medical or mental health professionals.

Acknowledgments

This book could not have been written without...

My clients throughout the years that have entrusted me for help. From them I have learned about the infinite potential of the human body. For their invaluable feedback and support, I am eternally grateful. They are the reason for A New BMI.

Paul, for believing in me and my work. For his willingness to help, even with those not-so-fun tasks, in order to make this book a reality. For his vision for A New BMI and his tireless devotion to its message. He is my inspiration.

Rangadevi, who keeps me true to myself and to my word. For offering me her best pair of listening ears every time I need them. For her commitment to my endeavors and for her friendship, I am truly blessed.

Kat, my patient, yet thorough editor who tidily cleans up the messes I manage to make. Her valuable input and careful eye contributed greatly to making A New BMI a much better read.

Dill, who showed me how to step through my fear of the unknown and just write the book already. Here it is!

" and i said to my body, softly.

' i want to be your friend.'

it took a long breath and replied,

' i have been waiting my whole life for this' "

Nayyirah Waheed

Table of Contents

A New BMI

Preface

I've been observing bodies in motion my whole life. I remember following the sport of gymnastics with a passion that I can barely put into words. As a child, I spent about as much time upside down as right side up. If gymnastics were on TV, I was right there, watching every move with rapt attention. Posted in my room were pictures of Lludmilla Tourischeva, Olga Korbut, and Cathy Rigby. I would do my very best to emulate what I saw them doing. I spent hours teaching my body how to do a front or back walkover. My father built a balance beam for me in the backyard so I could make believe I was an Olympian gymnast. I suppose I've never outgrown this fascination with moving the body.

As foreign a concept as this may seem to some, I have always welcomed the challenge of asking my body to try something new. For me, there's nothing quite like the feeling of accomplishment when your body takes over and says "yes, I can do this." It's quite extraordinary when you realize that the body has learned what you were willing to spend the time to teach it and you can now enjoy the freedom of allowing your body to move in new and extraordinary ways.

No wonder then that my first real job after graduating from Duke University in 1980 (yes, way back then) was to coach gymnastics. As a French major, I enjoyed my liberal arts education, but my heart was always drawn to helping the body move to its fullest potential. It didn't take long for me to realize that I could be a better coach if only I knew more about the human body and its performance potential.

After two years in graduate school in Biomechanics and another two years of graduate school in Exercise Physiology, I received my Master's degree in Health and Human Performance at East Carolina University and quickly assumed the role of Fitness Director at the Duke University Diet and Fitness Center. That was 25 years ago and I still recall how much I enjoyed helping people learn how to move their bodies by developing fitness programs for those whose body size had become a limiting factor to their participation in exercise programs.

Leaving Duke Diet and Fitness, I spent time as a personal trainer with my own private studio for a couple of years but was then called by Pritikin Longevity Center to serve as fitness director for their residential weight loss program in Miami. Two years in South Florida was enough for me, so I returned to Durham, North Carolina, where I served as fitness director, first for a local country club and then at Structure House, another residential weight loss center where I finally came to the conclusion that focusing on weight as the "issue" doesn't really meet the needs of those who suffer so greatly because of their body weight.

When it became evident to me that these centers made as much or more money from their return clientele as from their new enrollees, I began questioning my own role in perpetuating the diet and exercise myth. When I first began teaching how to lose weight by eating right and exercising, I was convinced that I was doing the right thing. However, my confidence waned as time went by, and I knew that there had to be a better way to promote health and fitness, one that didn't focus on body weight as the defining issue.

I believe that body size should not have to interfere with enjoyment of physical fitness. Without straying from that belief, I have changed my viewpoint about how to achieve fitness goals. Based upon my observations throughout my career in the health and fitness field, particularly in residential weight management programs, I have determined that the path to health and fitness can be accomplished without following the old rules. There is a better way.

Now I have confidence that my new approach is far closer to the truth and what the body needs to be healthy and perform as it should. My truth may seem a bit far-fetched to those who are convinced that body weight is the best reflection of optimal health, but I will explain what I have discovered to be a far better approach and one that meets a very different need than the achievement of weight loss.

Here I am, ready to speak my truth. This book is my effort to demonstrate how health cannot be measured by numbers on a scale but must be felt and experienced by the physical body. Until you are able to connect with your body and grow in your appreciation of what your body is capable of doing for you, your health and your body will suffer.

As long as you continue to define health with a tool as limited as body mass index, you will continue to fall short of the optimal health target. Where your attention goes reflects your personal values, convictions, and beliefs. When you focus on your weight, weight becomes your defining issue. If you really want to examine what's important to you, watch where you place your attention.

In Body Mind Intentions, my 8 week workbook which outlines a path to A New BMI, focus is placed upon maintaining and boosting energy levels, not on weight loss. As a gift to you, Lesson One of Body Mind Intentions is available simply by opting into my mailing list at anewbmi.com.

If the statement "That which you resist persists" is true, it only makes sense that we all continue to struggle with issues of body weight. We, as a nation, have waged war on obesity. Therefore, we have waged war on our own bodies. We are losing the battle of the bulge, yet we continue to practice the same methods (dieting) and get the same results (short-term success, long-term failure, and supreme frustration).

One definition of insanity is repeating the same behavior and expecting a different result. If you apply this to what we are experiencing in the war on obesity, our methods are bordering on levels of pure insanity.

It's time for a better way.

It's time to introduce A New BMI: Body Mind Intelligence.

Chapter One

**Good-bye, Body Mass Index —
Hello, Body Mind Intelligence**

It is time for A New BMI. It is time for a new marker of
health. It is time to introduce the concept of Body Mind
Intelligence. It is time to awaken to the wisdom of the
human body and learn to listen and respond. It is time to
pay attention when the body speaks. It is time to take the
most important step you can take on the road to achieving
optimal health.

The aim of Body Mind Intelligence is to help you live in a
better relationship with the body you have right here and
right now so that you are able to live in accordance with its
needs instead of just following the suggestions of the latest
online article or diet craze. This is the closest, most intimate
relationship you will ever have, and you are being called
upon to appreciate the marvelous creation that is your
physical self.

The human body is truly amazing. It is a vastly adaptable
and changeable creation. It is your home, your place of
being as you walk upon this earth. Your physical body is the
means through which you experience all the richness of life
and all the beauty this world has to offer. What you see and
what you feel both arise because you have a body.

Can you recall the most beautiful sunset you have ever
seen? Your body was there. Remember how it felt to hold

your newborn child for the very first time? Your body was there.

As you think about every single experience you have ever had since the moment of your birth, your body has been right there. You would not have had or been able to recall that experience without it. Seems pretty basic, but we all certainly do take it for granted.

The gift of life in the exquisite form of a physical body...

This body did not come to you with an owner's manual on how to best take care of, operate, or tend to it. Optimal performance of this incredible body of yours depends upon you to provide the care and maintenance necessary for your body. You learned from your parents and your school teachers how to take care of yourself when you were young. As you became an adult, you learned from others and from the information that was available to you to teach you about your health and wellness.

You rely upon books, magazines, media, the Internet, and most importantly your healthcare provider to give you good information. I don't believe any of you intend to become unhealthy. Most of you strive to live your life in such a way that you won't get sick and that you can enjoy independence and quality of life. Don't we all want to feel good and enjoy life?

If I were to ask what is the most important thing you can do for your health, I bet I would get a wide variety of answers. Eat well and exercise are right at the top of the list. But what exactly does it mean to eat well and exercise? Precisely... The confusion has begun. One day's "must do" becomes the next year's "must avoid." How are we supposed to figure it all out? Not even the so-called "experts" agree.

So what is the most important thing you can do for your health? Perhaps you would answer me with something along the lines of "maintain a healthy body weight." If I were to ask you what do you need to do if your body weight is more than it should be, most likely you would answer with "lose weight." And if I were to inquire how to lose weight, you would say "eat less and exercise more" or some other iteration of this same premise. Yes, of course—and the world is flat.

And if I asked what is the greatest threat to our nation's health?

Obesity or Ebola? Fat or fatigue? Too many calories or too much stress?

You get the idea. You are confused, and much of this confusion is due to our misunderstanding of the relationship between body weight and health and the story we've been told about what our weight is supposed to be.

No decent obesity conversation is complete without mention of body mass index (BMI), which has come to be accepted as the definitive measure of how well someone is doing with their weight relative to their height. The higher the BMI, the more at risk that individual's health is. That is what we accept as the truth about our weight. Yet, many do not even realize that the BMI was not intended to measure health, especially not for an individual. Time for a history lesson...

This widely used measurement was originally created by Adolphe Quetelet, a scientist in the 1800s, as a ratio to express the relationship of weight to height. The actual formula is as follows:

weight (kilograms) / height (meters squared)

In the 1970s, another scientist, Ancel Keys, mentioned the measure in his studies because he found it came the closest to body fat percentage, a measure of how much fat weight an individual carries relative to his total body weight. Keys warned that the body mass index, as he called it, was best utilized to measure populations as a whole, *not individuals*, as it cannot account for individual variations such as age, gender, race, or muscular build.

However, the National Institutes of Health (NIH) adopted the old BMI in 1985, and it became an easy standard for doctors to use in their practices to help identify patients who were outside the norm. In 1998, NIH consolidated the threshold for men and women, as well as establishing a BMI of 25–30 as "overweight" and over 30 as "obese." The numbers were relatively simple to use and have continued to serve as a definition of what constitutes a healthy body size as well as cut-off points for those who need treatment. How convenient and concise!

Because of the costs of medical conditions that are so closely associated with body weight, such as type 2 Diabetes, hypertension, and high cholesterol, there will most likely continue to be discussion in our medical community about the necessity of treating obesity. Requirements for bariatric surgery involve the inclusion of risk factors for disease in addition to the recommended BMI standards. I am not here to argue for or against medical intervention, but I am strongly urging all of us, physicians included, to view health through a different lens, not through that of an inadequate standard such as the old BMI.

A meta-analysis published by *JAMA* in January 2013 showed that the lowest risk of all-cause mortality belongs to those who have a BMI in the 25–30 range, which represents approximately 30% of females and 40% of males in the United States. Furthermore, although there was some increased risk of mortality in the grade 1 obesity (BMI 30–35) category, it was not as significant as the risks shown for higher rates of obesity, that is, a BMI classification of greater than 35. Almost half of adults in the United States who are classified as obese fall into the grade 1 category.

If you are following my reasoning, this evidence suggests that for a majority of Americans, the recommendation to lose weight cannot be based upon relative health risks because clearly the greatest risk is for the smaller minority who are classified under grade 2 (BMI > 35) or grade 3 (BMI > 40) obesity. I can see the benefit of preventing weight gain for health reasons but not necessarily the value of a recommendation of weight loss across the board.

There is strong evidence that other causal factors contribute to the health risks that are blamed on obesity. The greatest threat to our health is physical inactivity, not obesity. Cardiorespiratory fitness is one of the best predictors of longevity that we have, as shown by strong research published by Cooper Center Longitudinal Studies and led by Steven Blair, PhD.

A meta-analysis of fitness versus fatness on all-cause mortality was most recently published in *Progress in Cardiovascular Diseases*, Jan–Feb 2014. Compared to normal-weight fit individuals, unfit individuals had twice the mortality rate, regardless of BMI. Overweight and obese fit individuals were at no greater risk than normal-weight fit individuals, which leads to the recommendation of a focus on physical activity and fitness-based interventions rather than weight-loss-driven approaches to reducing mortality-based risk.

Despite what we know about physical activity and health, we still continue to pursue weight loss as the best action we can take for our health. In fact, it seems to be an obsession as we search for the best way to lose weight in order to enjoy optimal health.

If you are beginning to ask yourself why, then you are absorbing this information and drawing some conclusions, much like I have for many years. Now that I have some life experience to help me put things into perspective, I have begun to realize that when things just don't seem to add up or don't seem to make logical sense—*follow the money.*

The diet industry makes over $60 billion dollars a year, dependent upon your belief that weight loss is the path to health and happiness. As such, your desire to lose weight is propagated through their advertising and marketing. As long as you believe that you can be more beautiful, healthier, and more lovable at a smaller size than that at which you are right now, they have a greater likelihood of getting you to give them your money. The diet industry *loves* your money, and they care far more about *your money* than they do about you and *your health.*

I do care about you and your health. If I were in this for the money, I would need to guarantee you that Body Mind Intelligence leads to weight loss. I simply cannot and will not make that promise. I can promise you that adopting a New BMI can lead to significant, positive improvements in how you feel and how you move.

Even though I have taught exercise concepts related to body weight in some of the most reputable weight loss centers in the world and have written articles and books on exercise and weight loss, I am now fully aware that exercise alone is a very poor weight-management tool. Yes, exercise matters, but not in the manner we've been led to believe.

On top of the diet industry, there are plenty of others vying for your hard-earned cash. Think about it. The food industry, the pharmaceutical industry, dietary supplements— yes, even the health care industry needs to make sure you are ready to buy what they have to offer. These industries rely on your being "broken" and your belief that you need to be fixed. Your lack of health is money flow in their direction.

In whose best interest is it for you to be healthy? Yours, of course!

Let's return to our discussion of why we need a New BMI. Currently, when it appears that your body mass index puts you in the overweight or obese category, the first recommendation you receive is weight loss. Going on a diet is the next step—some combination of eating less and moving more. The problem is that 95% of those who lose weight through this method end up gaining back the weight. Only 5% of weight loss efforts are maintained in the long term, that is, for at least five years or beyond.

Can you imagine being prescribed a drug for a medical condition, whatever it may be, that will only temporarily relieve the symptom and also carries a risk of the condition coming back and being even more difficult to treat the next time? What if the doctor told you, "Here's this highly recommended drug I want you to take, but it really only works 5% of the time?" What would you want to say or do? Chances are, once you got over the urge to slap him or her, you would ask, "Isn't there something else that gets better results than that?"

Imagine being told that you could feel better, reduce your risk of death and disease, and have a greater quality of life as a result of this new approach. You may or may not lose any weight, but chances are very good you can prevent further weight gain. Does that sound any better to you? It certainly does to me.

Body Mind Intelligence offers you the opportunity to feel better, have more energy, enjoy a higher quality of life, manage stress, reduce your chance of dementia, and maintain your youthful vitality. Wow! Seriously? What is this stuff? Don't you want to try it?

You will find that the new BMI just makes good sense, as well as being based upon sound scientific evidence. The concept of Body Mind Intelligence has emerged from my determination and desire to create a new way to approach your health without focusing upon weight loss. It is my effort to put forth an alternative way of creating optimal health through a reasonable and achievable program of moving the body and quieting the mind.

Chapter Two

Say "I Do"

The body is an amazing creation. The human body is marvelous in its capacity to adapt and conform to whatever you ask of it. Exercising the body creates a demand, and the body adapts in order to meet that demand. I remain in awe of the performance potential of the human body.

The environment in which you live also creates a demand on the body, and the body again adapts accordingly. An example is the head position someone takes when texting. Typically, the head drops forward, and the upper back becomes rounded in order to focus on the screen of the phone. The more texting occurs and the more this particular movement is performed, the better the body will adapt to the demands of texting. The head will begin to drop forward and the shoulders round as gravity pulls against the weight of the head. Eventually, the body adapts by assuming a stooped posture. There's even a new medical term for this condition: text neck.

Text neck supports texting but does not support proper posture. Text neck also interferes with breathing, as it hinders your ability to take a full inhalation.

Sitting creates a different demand on the body. As the legs are bent at the hip, a shortening will occur at the front of the hip and thigh and in the back of the knee.

The more you sit, the more the body will accommodate the sitting posture, unfortunately at the risk of compromising your upright posture.

Fortunately, it is possible to counteract these negative adaptations through an intentional practice of moving the body in its natural patterns. I recommend taking an organic approach to moving your body, finding ways to challenge your body without inducing injury.

Use movements that are natural, varied, and at the level your body can manage. As a supplement to the first lesson in *Body Mind Intentions*, a workbook for health enhancement, I include an instructional video that teaches movement patterning. To take advantage of this gift, please visit my website and sign up for your introductory lesson.

It's online at www.anewbmi.com

Learning the limits of your body's capacity for movement requires you to connect with your body. That connection is a two-way conversation. You cannot just tell the body you want it to do a certain thing or move a certain way. You cannot expect your body to be there for you when you need it if you are not also asking the body what it needs in return.

Many exercise programs fail as a result of asking the body to do more than it has the capacity to handle or adapt. Your personal motivations play a key role as well. When you exercise, what is the end result you hope to achieve?

Do you view exercise as something you do "to" the body or "for" the body? Give this some serious thought because your health depends upon your answer. Contemplate your own motives for why you choose to exercise. Write down the top three reasons why you exercise or why you think you should exercise. Study them and see if your desires are more about changing your body or helping your body. Does your exercise program reflect you caring about how your body looks or how your body feels?

Is your desire to move centered on wanting your body to look a certain way or feel a certain way? Are you motivated based upon external factors or more internal factors? Do you think you are motivated intrinsically or extrinsically?

When you view exercise as something you do "to" the body, you are not allowing the body to be the active participant in the process. Some people view exercise only as a way to burn calories, and that is the only value it holds for them. That is an external point of view, an extrinsic motivator for moving the body. It separates you and your body.

Listening to your body is critical to your health and well-being and for tapping into your own Body Mind Intelligence. Listening to the body means you are paying attention to the messages the body sends to you in the form of feelings. It is easy for you to recognize feelings of hunger, thirst, and cold. Other feelings such as sadness or happiness are sometimes a bit more difficult to decipher.

Uncomfortable, negative feelings capture your attention as
you feel the need to "fix" them right away. Positive feelings
may be more elusive because they are subtle and do not
necessarily require you to act upon them; you enjoy them.

Sometimes your feelings make you so uncomfortable that you
want to avoid them. Perhaps you try to avoid them
altogether or deny that they even exist. Anxiety and fear can
stop you in your tracks, leaving you unable to move forward
or take any action at all.

Ignoring your feelings is your way of not paying attention to
your body and is the result when you continue to live in your
head. When you ignore your feelings or pretend they don't
exist, you are separating yourself from your body.

Feelings are the body's way of giving you information.
Feelings are signals from the body that are telling you what is
happening in your world. Feelings carry information.
Feelings are our bodies' way of talking with us, telling us
about our environment.

Feelings can sometimes seem overwhelming, but there is a
way to help you be more in control. Practicing mindfulness
allows you to see feelings as information, not as a threat.

In the practice of mindfulness, we observe but do not judge
those feelings or sensations. As soon as you judge or place a
meaning on them, each becomes an emotion with an
electrical charge attached to it. That charge can impact the

body positively or negatively depending upon how you label the feeling. That charge is carried throughout the nervous system and impacts every cell of your body.

Just as the environment creates adaptation in your body, so do your thoughts. Every single thought you have is registered in your body. Medical intuitive Carolyn Myss says, "Your biography becomes your biology." Everything that's ever happened to you is part of who you are, physically and emotionally.

How you think, how you feel, and how you move become who you are.

You cannot separate yourself from the body. It is who you are. Your physical body is the home for your heart and your soul. If you want the body to flourish and thrive, it depends upon you to listen and pay attention to the messages it sends to you every moment of every day.

In sickness and in health, so long as you both shall live... Say "I do" because you and your body are married. You and your body are in a permanent, long-term relationship.

When you consider all the elements that make a relationship work or fail, you may apply them to your relationship with your own body. Compassion and care, love and attention, forgiveness and communication—the list goes on and on. Perhaps you can come up with some yourself.

The key to any great relationship is communication. And the key to great communication is to learn how to listen, really listen. Try to understand what the body is telling you before you jump to conclusions or run away.

Pay close attention to the subtle signs and signals the body gives to you. Listen. Your body is speaking to you. When it speaks to you in a whisper and you don't hear it, it will speak louder. Eventually, in order to be heard, the body will scream its needs at you. That is the point when you are experiencing chronic pain or illness.

If you have ever had a health crisis of your own, there were most likely signs and signals from your body before it became a full-blown crisis. This is often the case when you choose to ignore the body and continue to push through in spite of fatigue or pain. A health crisis is the body's way of screaming "STOP!! I can't do this anymore!" If you ignore the body, it eventually will find a way to make you stop and pay attention.

You also need to cultivate compassion for your body. Appreciate your body for all that is does for you. Express your gratitude to your body. Practice forgiveness for any shortcomings your body may have because nobody (or no body) is perfect.

Trust your body and know that it wants what is best for you as well. Do you trust that your body is there for you?

Are you there for your body? Is it a mutually supportive
relationship?

Do you trust your body? Do you ever feel that you have
been betrayed by your body?

I have known many clients over the years who believed they
could not connect with their bodies. I have heard them say
that they actually feel "betrayed" by their bodies, that their
bodies will fail them, particularly as they attempt to begin a
program of exercise and movement.

If you do not trust your body, please consider that you hold
some degree of responsibility for that disconnection. Not
listening and separating yourself from the body can have a
negative impact on your relationship. When you stop
listening, when you disconnect from your feelings, when you
live from the neck up, your body and your health suffer.

Cultivating a relationship with your body means paying
attention when a feeling arises. When you feel tapped out,
start figuring out how to renew your energy resources. Begin
with getting enough sleep. Continue to find ways to move
your body and quiet your mind.

Connection with the body can occur in an almost infinite
variety of ways. I have discovered several methods that I
like and find helpful. You may want to try some of my
suggestions, or you may have some of your own.

How you make the connection is not nearly as important as the connection itself.

Spending time in the natural world allows you to be in a setting that takes you away from the distractions of the modern world and puts your body into an environment that feels just right. When entering the woods or watching a sunset, you are living in the moment, noticing the sights and sounds of what is unfolding right in front of you. Hiking in the woods is an activity that I enjoy on a regular basis. The walk becomes a natural means of moving through and appreciating the forest in all its beauty. The walking no longer "counts" as exercise but takes on a greater significance by feeding my soul.

Yoga is another way of connecting mind and body. The practice of yoga goes far beyond the boundaries of "exercise" and, when practiced as intended, puts you into a relationship of grace and gratitude for the body, here and now. Yoga is not about struggling to achieve but about learning your body's own limitations and potential. With regular yoga practice, you begin to notice how the body shifts and changes, that it is truly a reflection of your spirit.

If you love animals, as I do, you already know how they are able to help you relax and appreciate the moment. I have discovered that horses are especially suited to helping you connect with your body. Because horses rely entirely upon energetic connection as a means of communication, you must remain present and grounded in order to work with them in an effective manner.

I incorporate equine-facilitated learning into my teaching connection with the body and have found it to be very helpful to my clients who find it difficult to get "out of their heads" and "into their bodies."

Keeping a journal is also helpful as you can recognize feelings through the activity of writing. Writing with pen and paper engages your body in the process and allows you time to reflect. Reflection time should always include tuning into the sensations and feelings of your body.

Dancing is the full expression of your physical self. Everyone loves to dance. Every Body is a dancer. Dance is the celebration of life. Every time you move your body, you are dancing. Let every move you make be your celebration of life.

I also recommend that in order to connect with the body, you need to consciously disconnect from technology. When your attention is focused upon a device or screen, it cannot be focused upon the body. No wonder we are so "disconnected" from our bodies: we are too "connected" to our technology.

Take time to disconnect from the distractions. Take time to be with your body. If you go for a walk, remain completely focused upon being present with your body. Going for a walk outdoors and putting on earphones is just like sitting at the dining room table and talking on the phone while everyone around you would like for you to be with them. Your body wants you to be present so you can have a relationship.

Open the lines of communication. Stop shutting the body out by finding ways to connect with it.

Why not give yoga a try? How about dancing? Is there a sport or skill you would like to learn? When was the last time you rode a bike or a horse? The list can grow as long as you would like. It's all up to you how you want to cultivate your relationship with your body. Your body will thank you for it.

When you live in your head, your thoughts alone create your state of health. When you live in a healthy relationship with your body, your body reflects health back to you. From this day forward, you and your body will support each other for better or worse, for richer or poorer, in sickness and in health, so long as you both shall live.

Chapter Three

Something Old, Something New

Cultivate your relationship with your body through movement. Use slow, controlled, deliberate movements performed with attention to correct technique. Be present and focus on your body.

Our movement patterns, like our thought patterns, are developed over a lifetime. When you move incorrectly or don't move at all, the body accommodates and adapts to the environment you create for it and for the specific demands you place upon it.

To enjoy optimal physical health, you have to move your body. If, however, you have developed any strength imbalances in your musculoskeletal system or you have any limitations in your range of motion, you may have developed movement patterns that are not as functionally correct as they need to be. To correct the imbalance, you need to relearn what it is like to move organically and efficiently, to create less stress on your body.

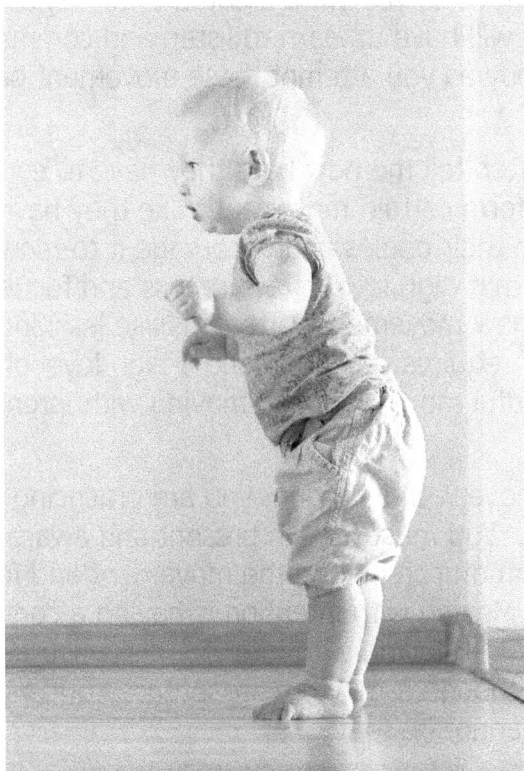

If you want to know what a correct movement pattern is like, simply observe a child. The spine is long and extended. The head balances beautifully on the vertebral column. A forward bend is created at the hinge of the hip, not in the mid-to-low back. Getting up and down from the floor is effortless as the child attempts his first steps.

Although it may seem foreign to you as you begin to relearn and reestablish correct movement patterning, you are

learning to move as you were created to move, as a child
moves. You will have to learn to listen and communicate
with your body as you attempt these movement patterns.

My clients often tell me how hard they have to concentrate in
order to perform certain moves. It's like they have to wake
up a place in their bodies and encourage it to move.
Maintaining that high level of awareness and focusing upon
performing new movement patterns is like learning a brand
new skill. It requires repetition and a high level of attention.
I call it "mindful movement" or "moving with intention."

When you move with intention, you are practicing
mindfulness. You must remain present and aware, focusing
your attention on completing the movement and feeling the
movement. Moving with intention is having a conversation
with your body. Moving with intention asks you to be
engaged. Although it may require intense concentration, the
movement cannot be forced.

It is also important to maintain variety in movement patterns,
as it is possible to injure yourself by repeating the same
movement over and over again. Always keep in mind that
repetitive motion is the primary cause of exercise-related
injury. When practicing moving with intention, you want to
vary your movements and think of the body as a whole,
rather than isolated parts.

Pain and injury also result from imbalances in the
musculoskeletal system. In relearning movement patterns,
you are attempting to correct some of those imbalances, but

remember that you are especially vulnerable to injury when trying new and unaccustomed patterns.

Pain is the primary reason most people avoid exercise. The fear of the pain returning or getting worse keeps people immobilized. That's completely understandable. If the knee is painful, it certainly makes sense that you would want to avoid anything that makes it worse.

It is possible, though, to move up to and around the pain itself. If you are listening carefully and paying attention to feedback from the body, you may be able to improve or increase the amount of movement before you experience pain. This is the marvelous adaptability of the human body.

Your environment creates many of the imbalances in the body, the best example being too much sitting. As discussed earlier, your body adapts to the sitting position, making it more difficult to stand up or walk about.

If I could put everything I know about exercise physiology into one single statement, it would be this. The more you ask your body to move, the greater the chances it will continue in its ability to move. The more you choose to sit still, the greater the chances that your body will not be able to stand back up.

Your lesson: keep moving.

As a special gift for you, I am offering Lesson One of *Body Mind Intentions*, a workbook I developed to help you incorporate physical activity and mindfulness into your day-to-day life. As you may realize by now, I like to focus upon organic, natural movements.

Some examples are available in the supplemental video that I offer as a special gift for you, along with the first lesson of the workbook.

Just go online to my website at www.anewbmi.com

Chapter Four

The Big Disconnect

So now you know—you cannot measure health by stepping on the scale. Nor can you measure your self-worth in pounds. Have you ever been put in a bad mood after finding out you've gained weight? Face it, we all have.

Many years ago, when I was still in college, I obsessed over the scale. I would weigh myself, then go pee and poop, and weigh myself again—because it was never good enough. I wanted my body to look a certain way, and I completely restricted my food intake to maintain that ideal. I managed to keep that low weight for approximately one year, regained the lost weight plus twenty more pounds. I was miserable. Regardless of how much I weighed, I wasn't happy.

I know I am not alone. Many of us strive to lose weight to feel better about our bodies and about ourselves. It's a never-ending chase of an unattainable dream. It's a mirage of smoke and mirrors, keeping us on a perpetual quest that has no end point.

"You can never be too rich or too thin." We might find this statement amusing, but it certainly sums up our culture in one simple phrase. One of the best ways to get attention is to say you know how to accumulate wealth or lose weight and are willing to share your secrets. It's also an awesome money maker!

By the way, just because someone drives a luxury vehicle does not mean they are rich. You just can't tell by looking. The car you drive is not in direct correlation to your monetary worth. Nor is having a body closer to what is considered the "ideal."

Having a body that is above "ideal" weight says nothing about your moral character, your eating habits, or your state of health.

Our cultural obsession with thinness coupled with the near impossibility of weight loss creates a no-win situation, leading to epidemic numbers of people feeling dissatisfied with their bodies. And it doesn't stop there—now our children are attempting diets because of their fear of being called "fat."

The primary reason children are bullied is body weight. Name calling, teasing, and exclusion leave lasting impressions and result in poor self-esteem and declining academic performance. Furthermore, bullying increases the risk of suicide in addition to a multitude of health issues that follow them right into adulthood.

Weight bias has far-reaching consequences. There is ample scientific evidence to show that overweight people face discrimination in employment, education and healthcare, having a significant impact on their economic, social, mental and physical well-being. Research from the Yale Rudd Center for Food Policy and Obesity (now UConn Rudd Center) reveals that adult overweight women frequently experience weight bias from their health care providers. Their research reveals that physicians view their obese patients as less compliant and less self-disciplined, resulting in their finding it less desirable to help the overweight patient. Considering how much weight bias exists in our medical community, it is entirely possible that some of the health risk factors associated with being overweight are due to lack of the same standard of care. And considering that many overweight patients will avoid going to their doctors because they feel shamed by them or they want to avoid the scale, we must look at the health consequences of obesity in a different light.

As an advocate for physical activity and for the human body, I find it disconcerting how many people I encounter who avoid moving their bodies simply because of the fear of being stigmatized. I wish I had a solution to offer that could take away the blame and shame placed on individuals simply as a result of their body size. What I can do, however, with A New BMI, is present methods of moving and enjoying the body that transcend the old paradigms about body weight. It is possible to achieve health and feel better in your body without feeling shame or guilt. Body Mind Intelligence offers a new path for your health and well-being.

It becomes obvious that weight bias and stigma contribute to the stress experienced by those who seek to lose weight because they are convinced that they are broken, that there is something wrong with them that needs to be fixed. Their stress leads to binging and further weight gain—certainly not the "hoped-for" result. As it is also well documented that stress leads to negative health consequences, we can also draw a conclusion that the stress of weight bias may be responsible for the health consequences of obesity rather than the weight itself.

I offer up these observations with the specific intention that we begin to view those who struggle with their weight from an entirely different perspective. While I cannot change society, I assert that it is possible to make positive, impactful changes in an individual's health simply as a result of moving the body and quieting the mind.

Since we can all agree that learning how to manage stress results in positive health outcomes, I propose a new standard for measuring health, something other than the bathroom scale.

At any moment of any day, you determine how energetic you feel. You have your own innate sense of your energy level.

Imagine your energy level is much like a fuel gauge on your car. You can feel "full": energetic, enthusiastic, and ready for anything. Or you can feel "empty": depleted and lethargic. And of course, anything in between. We will call this tool the Vim Index (VIMDEX), a self-measured feeling of available energy.

VIMDEX: How much energy do I have _right now?_

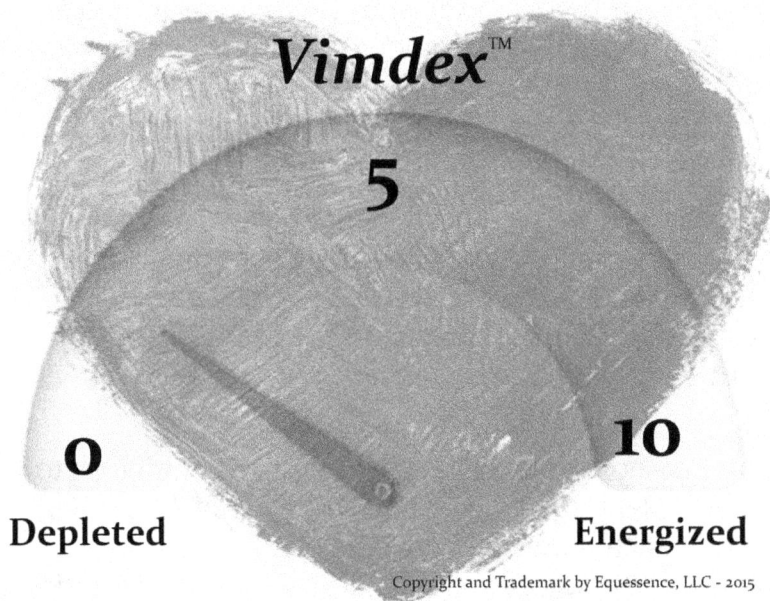

Vimdex™

5

0   10

Depleted   **Energized**

Your level of energy to go about your day-to-day life is certainly a better reflection of your health and well-being than stepping on a bathroom scale. And the amazing coincidence is that many of the factors that contribute to weight gain are the very same factors that leave you feeling depleted:

- Stress
- Lack of sleep
- Poor nutrition
- Dehydration
- Medications
- Poor physical fitness

Instead of focusing upon body weight as your measure of success, focus upon improving your **Vimdex**. To have more energy to go through your day, you must take action to identify where your energy goes and how to get it back.

As you seek to do what you can to replenish your energy stores, two important and immediate actions you may take are moving the body and quieting the mind. That is why physical activity and mindfulness are the cornerstones of A New BMI: Body Mind Intelligence.

Although I acknowledge that proper nutrition contributes to health and well-being, it will not be the focus of A New BMI. In my experience from working in the diet industry, food quickly becomes the focus for change, often to the exclusion of other lifestyle factors. The clients at each of the residential weight loss programs where I served for so many years were already quite knowledgeable about their nutrition. Food was their focus and their fix. They were convinced they were "broken" and food was the reason why.

The "dieters" I worked with paid thousands of dollars weekly to gain control over food. I couldn't help but wonder whether they were enrolled in the programs to learn how to manage their body weight or to hide out where meals were provided so that they could give control of their food over to the program rather than take that responsibility for themselves. They were willing to pay for the safety of the program because they could not trust themselves.

I recall how many of the dieters would say "just tell me what to do." Their sincere need to have someone else tell them what they could not do for themselves both mystified and saddened me. And as long as they remained "on program," most were very successful at losing weight, sometimes as much as 10% of their body weight in four weeks' time—until they went back home, where things fell apart. Next thing you know, they were back "on program."

The more I observed these behaviors, the more I convinced myself that the best diet and exercise counseling in the whole wide world was not what these "dieters" needed. The evidence against dieting presented itself to me in the context of "obesity treatment." These programs (Duke, Pritikin, and Structure House) are the world's best at offering comprehensive care for treating obesity, each offering behavioral therapy, nutrition and fitness education along with medical supervision. If these programs were not able to help people keep the weight off, then what gives?

Furthermore, as the evidence against dieting mounted, as research continued to point to the restriction of calories leading to reduction in metabolic rate as well as to eating-disordered behaviors, I became increasingly uncomfortable with my role in perpetuating the diet-and-exercise paradox.

What I had noticed all along became even more apparent. In the dieters, I saw dissatisfaction, disconnection, and disease. They "hated" their bodies. They did not trust their bodies or themselves. Many told me they felt that their bodies had "betrayed" them. They suffered from a wide list of physical ailments. And they saw exercise as something they needed to do "to" their bodies, rather than "for" their bodies.

Those desperately seeking to lose weight found it difficult to engage in their bodies long enough to actually feel the difference it made to move. Many were far more focused on how many calories they could burn (again, a disconnected way to make exercise about food) than on finding enjoyment from connecting to their own bodies.

Exercise time in these residential programs was media time or telephone time or even work time. It was impossible to have a workout area without a television going or music blasting. "I need the distraction so I can go longer" was the given reason why.

At Pritikin, I recall big-screen televisions, two to three on each wall surrounding the cardio area, which held 30 treadmills. Everyone had their choice from a wide variety of channels. I specifically recall September 11, 2001, when I witnessed the devastation of the Twin Towers on each and every screen surrounding the cardio room.

Difficult as it was to absorb the event, having the image so clearly embedded in my psyche clearly created trauma in my own body, as I could not possibly escape my participation as a witness many times over. And every time that footage played across the television screen, we were all forced to relive the event.

As you become fully aware that your body cannot tell the difference between what is real and what is simply imagined, you can understand the negative impact your exposure to the "news" can have upon your body. The destruction of September 11 lives in all of us, and we carry that memory in our bodies.

I have observed the exercise "disconnect" phenomenon not only in the residential weight loss centers where I worked but also in widespread existence elsewhere. All health clubs have televisions in the cardio area. People read and fiddle with their phones while riding the recumbent cycles. Earphones are the norm.

Be honest—why do you want the distraction from the activity? This kind of "disconnect" occurs more frequently in workout facilities than outdoors, although I do see some people out on the trail with earphones attached. If you are to be fully present to the activity, you cannot be paying attention to your entertainment and to your body at the same time.

Perhaps not paying attention to the body is exactly what you are trying to accomplish. What does that disconnect have to do with Body Mind Intelligence? Body Mind Intelligence establishes that the path to health begins with being aware of and paying attention to the physical body. If you are guilty of exercise disconnect, you may want to explore your own motivations in tuning out the body in order to tune in to something else.

Chapter Five

Stepping Away from the Pain

If you want to feel better, consider these two things: Are you *moving* your body? What are you *thinking* about your body?

These two questions are closely related. How you answer them reveals why you may or may not have the energy and enthusiasm for life that you desire. If you are not moving your body and you are thinking negatively, it follows that your health may be suffering as a result. Being positive in outlook and taking the opportunity to move your body are two of the best actions you can take to feel better *right now*.

Trust comes from a positive mindset. Trust requires faith that your body is capable of taking care of you and is able to perform as needed for you. For many, the primary reason for not moving the body is lack of trust. Stemming from a fear associated with moving the body and rooted deeply in the subconscious is the belief that you cannot trust your body.

If you think you are about to experience something unpleasant, you are not likely to follow through with it. If you cannot trust your body to move without pain, it seems logical that there would be a great deal of resistance to exercise. If you have pain with exercise, you are not alone. If you have fear that you will do something wrong and hurt yourself, your concerns are valid.

I bring you good news! Quite often, correcting your movement patterns is enough to help alleviate or eliminate the pain. And certainly, moving the body correctly, with balance and efficiency, prevents injury.

Up until now, you may have heard that walking is great exercise. The belief is that walking is easy and anybody can do it. The problem you may have run into is that walking is not easy and your body cannot handle it. You are left feeling discouraged and frustrated as a result.

Walking is repetitive motion. As easy as it may seem to just go for a walk, if you have any musculoskeletal imbalances, even a simple walk can lead to a painful end. The most likely cause of your injury is overuse—repeating a pattern over and over until something fails. The body is no different than any structural system: if you place a demand beyond what it can handle, it will fail, most likely at the weakest point or at the point of greatest force or impact.

Perhaps you have had this experience already. You start a walking program for all the right reasons, and bam! Before you know it, something hurts. It could be your back, your knees, your hips, or your feet. Or perhaps you decided to try weight lifting and within just a few months, you start feeling a little something in your shoulder, elbow, or wrist...

Body Mind Intelligence offers you a new way of moving your body to help you avoid injury and pain.

Begin by changing your mind about your body. Instead of viewing everything as "exercise," focus upon the movement itself. Learn functional and easy patterns that will help you improve your strength, flexibility, and balance without injuring yourself.

Fear of moving the body is the single greatest barrier I've encountered in all these years of teaching and guiding people through movement and exercise. Sometimes the fear is around physical pain. Sometimes the fear is around painful feelings that arise when moving the body. Those feelings come from thoughts or emotions that manifest in the body. And the pain is just as real as it is from any musculoskeletal injury.

As an exercise physiologist, I've experienced the frustration of not knowing how to overcome this resistance that so many have to moving their bodies. I've preached the glories of physical fitness, and even with the knowledge of all the health benefits of exercise, there are those who remain "un-moved." Which begs the question so many of us ask when confronted with someone else's behavior that just doesn't add up: "what are they thinking?"

Ta-DA! That's it! Thoughts elicit feelings, and those feelings reside in the body. If your thoughts about your body are negative, moving your body only brings about negative, unpleasant feelings.

Positive thoughts create positive feelings, which leads to positive behaviors when it comes to moving your body. If you view your body positively, moving your body is no longer an activity to be avoided, but to be pursued. Moving your body is essential to your health and well-being. Thinking positive thoughts about your body makes it easier to be physically active.

Many of the negative thoughts people have about their bodies arise as a direct result of their beliefs about size and weight. Those negative beliefs prevent them from enjoying optimal health and well-being through physical activity. What you think impacts your movement potential and your health.

Every thought you have carries an electrical charge that is received and stored by every cell of your body. Therefore, your memories are stored not just as images in the mind but as feelings in the body. You cannot separate your thoughts and feelings from your body. The two are inextricably intertwined.

Body Mind Intelligence refers to all the information that our bodies are constantly receiving and processing. We have the five receiving senses of seeing, hearing, touching, tasting, and smelling. We also have a receiving sense that collects information through vibration, picking up on the flow of energy that surrounds us—sometimes referred to as our sixth sense.

In addition to picking up information for us, your body must process the information it receives. Your nervous system, including the brain, interprets the information it receives and then responds back to your body for appropriate action. Your fight-or-flight response is a perfect example of Body Mind Intelligence in action.

Because your basic survival mechanism is to fight or flee when you sense danger, your body prepares by signaling the adrenals to produce cortisol and adrenaline. Whether the danger is real or imagined, you get the same hormonal response in your body. Over time, excessive production of these stress hormones can be your physical downfall, leading to poor health outcomes such as diabetes, heart disease, and cancer.

Your body also prepares your muscles for fight or flight, most often showing up in the form of raising the shoulders in a defensive posture. Over time, this muscular tension becomes ingrained and interferes with your movement and your breathing. Tightness in the neck and shoulders reflects a chronic fight-or-flight response. If you find yourself grabbing the nape of your neck and rocking your head to the side, you are experiencing tension. Are you experiencing stress? Chances are...yes, indeed.

What you *think* becomes how you feel and how you move. What you experience, even in your mind's eye, manifests in your body.

The placebo effect is a perfect example of your mind influencing your body and your health. The *belief* that it will work is how sugar pills can have the same effect as real medicine.

Here's an example of the powerful influence the mind can have over your body. Alicia Crum, PhD, is a research psychologist who studies mind-set and its influence on the body. A recent study published in *Health Psychology* in July 2011 shows how mind-set can influence hunger and satiety. In this study, every subject drank the same 380-calorie milkshake on two separate occasions; however on one occasion they were told it was a "sensible" 140-calorie milkshake, and on the other occasion, subjects were told it was an "indulgent" 620-calorie milkshake.

Dr. Crum then measured what happened to ghrelin levels in response to drinking the milkshake. Ghrelin is a hormone produced in the gut that impacts our appetite. Called the "hunger hormone," it is released to stimulate food-seeking behavior. If the hunger is satisfied, ghrelin levels are decreased and food seeking behavior is reduced.

The outcome to this fascinating study was that following the ingestion of the "indulgent" shake, or what subjects believed to be the 620-calorie shake, ghrelin levels were three times lower than when they believed that they had just consumed a "sensible" 140-calorie milkshake. The psychological *belief* impacted the physiological *response*. Their belief about how satisfied they should feel following a low-calorie versus a high-calorie milkshake was reflected by hormone production in the gut.

Your mind has a powerful influence on your body and your health.

Hunger is a feeling from the body. Thirst is as well. What about sadness? Or anger? Are they feelings you have in your body or are they just thoughts? Chances are if there is a sensation that occurs in your body, you interpret it a certain way when you feel it. Just like hunger feels a certain way, sadness or happiness may also feel a certain way. Your emotions manifest as feelings in your body.

Every thought you have manifests in the body in one form or another. You cannot separate yourself from your thoughts and feelings, although you really do try. If you feel something unpleasant, your nature is to avoid it. It is the avoidance of those undesirable feelings that makes you want to shut down and cut yourself off from your body.

Many people live in their heads, completely absorbed in thought and not paying attention to what is happening right in front of them—and certainly not paying attention to the subtle messages their bodies are sending them all the time.

I spent many years working in residential obesity treatment programs, and I observed behaviors that reflect a disconnectedness from the body. First and foremost, I would listen to what people were saying about their bodies. The language of disconnection sounded like "I don't even recognize my body," "It feels like my body belongs to someone else," "I hate my body," "I have to lose the weight," "I wish I didn't have to exercise," and "My body has betrayed me."

These phrases were common. I heard similar language repeated in many different forms, but the sentiment was very much the same. The body had become a separate entity to be dealt with, far from being appreciated and loved.

I cannot wave a magic wand that makes people love their bodies. That hatred and separation from their bodies has occurred as a result of a belief system that hinders them in the pursuit of feeling better and enjoying optimal health. Focusing on body weight as something that "has to go" or viewing the body as something vile instead of holy can only lead to a loss of valuable energy and vitality.

How much energy do you expend chasing after the idea of having a different body? What do you think is the potential impact of that mind-set?

If you resist moving the body, the potential outcome is not being able to move. The more the body remains at rest, the more difficult it is to resist gravity. The more you choose to move the body, the easier movement becomes. It happens as a result of physical laws but also in direct response to your thoughts and beliefs.

Your body is a wonderful creation and deserves your care, attention, and respect. If you are interested in living a healthy, fulfilling life, your feelings about your body must become positive and nurturing. Body Mind Intelligence reflects a positive mindset and a healthy relationship with the physical self.

The purpose of this book is to educate, enlighten, and inspire a change from the current attitudes and beliefs about body weight and health and to move towards a greater awareness of how the mind influences the body.

The new BMI promotes health as it relates to the relationship between the body and the mind, not between height and weight, opening up the possibility that it is possible to achieve optimal health without focusing upon weight loss.

The new BMI teaches that caring for the body requires the maintenance of a positive attitude and the ability to listen and pay attention to the needs of the body, cultivated through physical activity and the practice of mindfulness. This is Body Mind Intelligence.

Chapter Six

Move Your Body

When you think about moving your body, what kind of emotional reaction do you have? What kind of feelings does the word "exercise" elicit from you? When you visualize your body in motion, what do you see and feel?

The feelings you have regarding your body have everything to do with your health. Body Mind Intelligence is the knowledge that your emotions guide your actions and your body is the reflection of your thoughts, feelings, and beliefs.

Somewhere along the way, in your pursuit of a "better body," you may have lost your appreciation for the body you possess. If your body doesn't look the way you desire, what kinds of thoughts or feelings do you have about that? Those negative thoughts impact your own health and well-being.

Your thoughts about moving your body may also be more negative than positive. What do you feel when you think about exercise? Take a moment and explore how your feelings may be interfering with your desire to move.

Your beliefs about exercise prevent you from the enjoyment of moving your body.

First of all, there are lots of rules and recommendations about exercise that are both confusing and confounding.

As an exercise physiologist, I am expected to know the answers about how many minutes, how many days per week, what intensity, what heart rate, what distance, how far, how high, how fast, and so on. I am proud of my career helping people realize their fitness potential. I have an extensive working knowledge of what it takes to achieve physical fitness. At the same time, I realize that the potential and capacity of every "body" is different. Sometimes the rules that work for one person do not create the same benefits in another.

Although the rules and guidelines may differ from one individual to the next, one fact remains. You were born to move.

Your capacity to move is nearly limitless. You need only admire the skill and grace of an accomplished athlete to just begin to realize the potential of the human body. We were all born with the capacity to move, but because we are no longer required to move as we were intended to by design, we lose that capacity.

The more you sit, the more your moving capacity is diminished. The more you move, the greater your potential to continue to move.

Observe a young child at play and realize that within you is that same capacity for movement and joy. You may have lost your ease of movement, but you have not lost your capacity. You may have lost your joy of movement, but you have not lost the need.

The human body requires movement to function. The diaphragm moves so you can breathe. Bowels move, the heart beats, and blood flows. Physical movement is the foundation of life. Even the process of procreation requires movement.

Your musculoskeletal system constantly moves in relationship to the pull of gravity, shaping you to the environment in which you live. Your relationship with gravity and moving against gravity is what keeps your body at its current functional capacity. The more you sit, the more your body takes on the shape of your seat, with just the right amount of tension to keep you from falling out of the chair.

The more you choose to move about in a variety of ways, the more accommodating the body becomes. The more sedentary you are and the less you move your body against gravity, the less your body is able to maintain its capacity to move and function.

Growing older is not to blame. Not moving is the culprit when you lose your stamina, strength, flexibility, and balance.

Your relationship with gravity starts at birth. As your body develops, you continue to learn how to move with gravity, and your muscles and bones strengthen to meet increasing demands. As you grow older, or more specifically, as you become less active, the body loses bone and muscle mass. Your metabolic rate drops, and fat accumulates.

When the body moves, stretching and tensing against gravity, all those negative changes can be prevented and even reversed. Your neuromuscular system responds, and you are able to do more, with greater strength, balance, and coordination.

If you approach moving your body with the curiosity of a child, you will begin to have the appreciation of what your body is capable of doing, rather than being angry or sad because of what you have lost. Your body adapts beautifully to whatever you ask, as long as you approach it with patience, kindness, and grace.

How does it feel when you get pushed at work beyond what you have the capacity to handle? How well do you perform if someone like your boss is telling you that you don't have a choice in the matter—do it or else? Do you feel any resistance to that approach? Would you prefer to have your boss ask you what you think you would need in order to complete the task? Your body feels the same way.

Your body has its own ways of telling you when it cannot handle what you're asking of it. If you think about it, you may already know little signs or symptoms that your body gives you that say "enough already!"

I know when I feel stressed and I'm pushing myself to get something done, my body talks back to me. I get little twitches and spasms that come and go, just letting me know that whatever it is I'm doing, my body is beginning to feel tapped out. For example, my eye twitches when I don't get enough sleep because I'm staying up late to finish a project. Sometimes when I am working on a dance move that I really want to learn, I do it over and over until I get it. Then later that day or the next day, I get this little tiny wiggle somewhere in my thigh. Just a little spasm, not painful, but just annoying enough so that I pay attention and rest as needed.

Chances are you have experienced delayed onset muscle soreness, one of the consequences of asking more of your body than it is accustomed to doing, a perfect example of your body adapting to a demand. The demand causes disruption of the muscle cell, and the body responds through the inflammatory process. Your soreness is a sign that your body is healing and getting stronger. A little bit of soreness is to be appreciated, not avoided. If, however, you experience soreness that is so painful that you find it difficult to move, that is a message from the body. It is letting you know that it is trying to get stronger for you, but this time you pushed too hard, exceeding your body's ability to heal and adapt.

Unfortunately, the loss of connection with your body makes it more difficult to know your own physical limitations and potential. This lack of knowledge of your own body leads to injury, pain, and suffering. Many well-intended exercise programs come to an abrupt halt because the body reaches its limit and pain becomes the only way it has to make you stop and pay attention.

When I am working with my clients, I ask them to pay close attention to this feedback from the body. Sometimes their bodies react immediately to a specific movement. That reaction could be pain. It could also be compensation in another area, as sometimes the body resorts to "cheating," that is, using a different muscle pattern to try and perform the movement. In other words, sometimes the message is delayed and shows up in a different part of the body.

My role as a trainer and movement educator is to be an advocate for the body, to be able to recognize messages from the body that even the client may not recognize. This is why I am a stickler for correct technique. It is not enough to just go through the motions: you need to learn correct patterning of the movement.

Because my approach to movement promotes connection with the body, there exists less likelihood of overdoing it. Even the smallest increases in movement make a positive difference while you and your body learn together your limitations and your potential.

If you know you are the all-or-nothing type, you will find the new BMI a refreshing difference from the way you have approached your body in the past. It is such a temptation to believe that if a little is good, a whole lot more should be better. When it comes to your body, a little can go a very long way. Doing more than the body can accommodate leads to injury and a prolonged recovery.

Finding the right balance between too much and too little can be frustrating to the average everyday exerciser. I've spent years teaching movement and encouraging physical activity. I learn something new nearly every time I approach the body. I can understand the frustration that you may have, not being able to determine what is best for you and your body.

There are lots of rules and regulations when it comes to exercise. Body Mind Intelligence requires you to set your own rules. Your body is different than anyone else's, and just because you've read or heard that you need to lift weights two times a week doesn't mean that is what your body can handle.

My frustration with the fitness community comes from something I myself was guilty of doing for many years. As an exercise physiologist, I had to know the "rules." I was the expert on heart rate, intensity, duration, blah blah blah. I made sure that I taught the rules correctly.

My clients and their bodies have taught me to go against the rules because the rules don't necessarily work for them. Perhaps you have found the same to be true for you. Perhaps you have done everything you know to be right but still are in pain or just aren't seeing any benefit. How frustrating is that?

Take heart, because you are going to discover your own set of rules for you and your body. You just have to be willing to listen and pay attention to your body and see how it responds when you ask it to move.

Being physically active is the single greatest predictor of longevity and quality of life. Move. A little today, maybe a little more tomorrow. Just move. As you spend more time in conversation with your body, it will tell you exactly what it needs.

Be inspired to move.

It is your birthright.

It is your opportunity to discover the limits and potential of your marvelous body.

Chapter Seven
Energy in Balance

You are now aware of just how much influence your thoughts have over your body and your health. You are also well aware of how physically exhausting it can be to deal with stressful events. Worrisome thoughts can also deplete your energy.

If you feel tired and lack energy, perhaps you are emotionally drained. Our negative, worrisome thoughts actually require our energy in order for us to give them our attention. Every time you revisit a stressful event, your body records it physically—whether or not that event is happening in real time or in your imagination. All emotion, whether positive or negative, is held by the body.

Remember the fuel gauge that describes how much energy we possess? Here's a figure that demonstrates how our bodies react to emotion and to movement in terms of energy balance.

Notice how negative recurring thoughts require energy and drain your fuel tank. Notice how bouts of moving the body and resting the body (recovery) serve to restore energy to the fuel tank. Also note how positive emotion, while it does not cancel the negative, can help decrease the impact of the negative over time. A mindfulness practice restores energy balance by lessening the emotional charge associated with thoughts and beliefs.

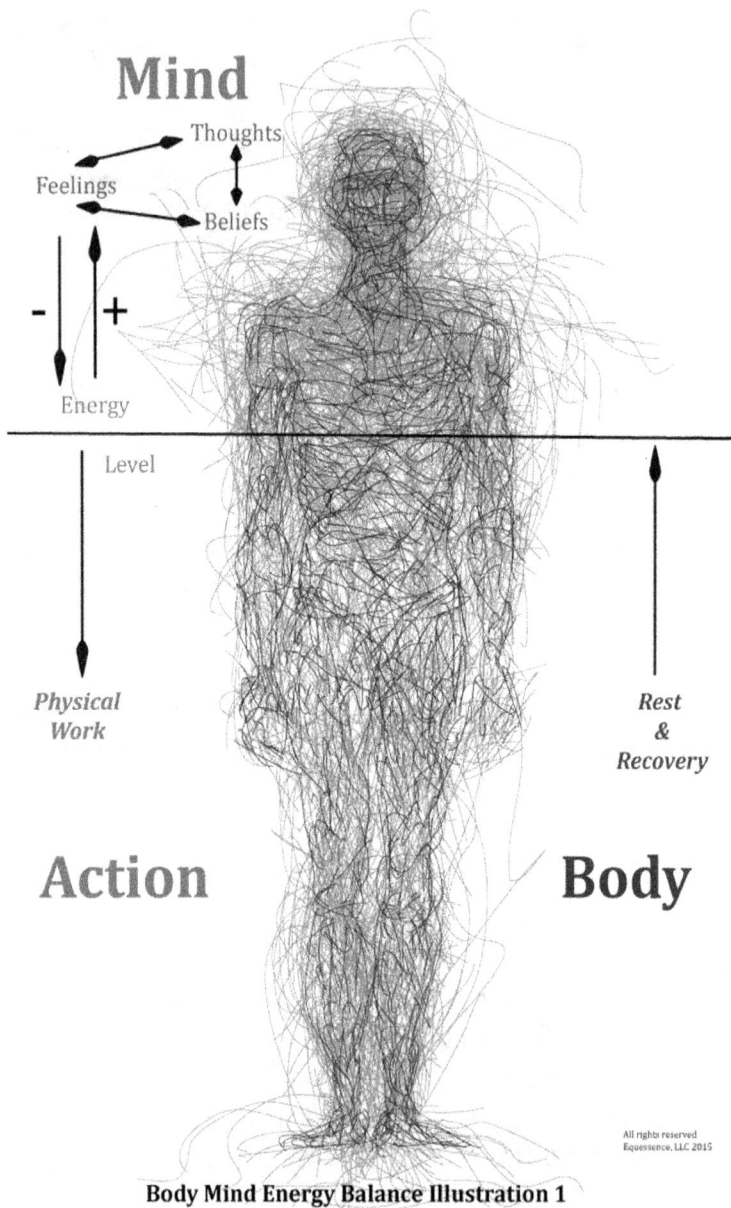

Mind

Thoughts

Feelings

Beliefs

− +

Energy

Level

Physical
Work

Rest
&
Recovery

Action

Body

Body Mind Energy Balance Illustration 1

I readily admit that there are other factors that are vital to your energy stores, such as nutrition and sleep. In no way am I able to cover all the issues that contribute to fatigue as I write this book, but please keep in mind that paying attention to the signs and signals that your body sends out to you can help you begin to address the needs of your body before your energy stores are depleted and your health begins to spiral downward. As you come to know your body better, you realize exactly what you and your body need to remain healthy. You will take the positive steps necessary to keep you and your body functioning at optimal levels.

Body Mind Intelligence arises from nurturing the relationship between you and your body. Having Body Mind Intelligence raises your awareness to how your thoughts impact your body and your health.

My approach to health encourages physical activity combined with the practice of mindfulness. As shown in our illustration on the previous page (Illustration 1), you must find a balance between moving the body and quieting the mind. Although you will experience improved health by incorporating one or the other into your life, optimal impact is achieved by creating a balance between the practices of movement and mindfulness.

The energy you need for living and thriving is your vitality. Your vitality is a reflection of your mental and physical vigor, your capacity to handle the challenges of day-to-day living. Maintaining and improving your vitality requires recognition of where you expend energy as well as what restores it.

Moving the body, although it requires energy output, enhances energy stores by allowing your body to become more physically fit. Your ability to do any kind of physical work depends upon your physical capacity, and your capacity is determined by what you actually do or don't do. Use it or lose it!

Quieting the mind requires effort on your part but results in less drain on your energy stores. Be aware of how your thoughts manifest in your body and what contributes to your feelings of fatigue. Having Body Mind Intelligence helps you realize that the energy you have to give to the demands of your life is a perfect reflection of your thoughts as well as your actions.

There are no rules other than determining what is best for you and your body. With my clients, what we do each session changes because the body shifts and changes. The body is made up of water. It only makes sense that it has fluid properties.

The reason I call myself a body advocate is because after so much experience working with different bodies, I realize that not only are no two individuals alike but no two days are alike. It is my role to help my clients recognize messages from the body so that all movements are performed appropriately. I act on behalf of the body, especially if the clients do not feel comfortable determining what the body can or cannot handle for themselves.

Quite often people have the expectation that the role of the personal trainer is to tell them what exercises to do and how to do them. Although such an approach can result in positive changes, it is necessary to be mindful of how the body responds. Through careful observation of my clients' movements and how their bodies respond, I gauge what is appropriate by learning their limitations through feedback from the body. Sometimes the feedback is in the form of discomfort or pain. Other times I will observe compensatory movement that also indicates that a limitation exists and must be recognized.

A concern I have about some of the personal trainers I have observed is how they focus on sets, reps, and numbers and not on the client. Many of my clients come and work with me because they have experienced injury and/or pain while with another trainer who either did not recognize the limitations of the client or lacked knowledge of correct movement technique.

I teach how to recognize and shift your movements based upon how the body responds. This process requires personal participation in the process of learning how to move your body correctly and how to adjust to what the body tells you. This combination of practicing awareness while moving the body is one aspect of developing your Body Mind Intelligence. As you grow in awareness, you improve your relationship with your body and learn how to respond appropriately to what it needs from you.

I love it when my clients tell me how they themselves determined what felt best for them or for their bodies based on their own assessment. And when I see them making their own adjustments for any given movement or exercise to accommodate their own limitations, it gets me so excited.

Having the ability to discern what your body needs and how you can accommodate for it, means far more than the ability to run farther or lift more. True mastery is the ability to communicate with your physical body. True mastery happens when you learn to pay attention to the body and focus upon what it is telling you.

Once true mastery is achieved, there is no longer a need to ask how much, how long, or how far. With true mastery, you are able to know yourself what your body can handle and how much you can ask of it.

Of course, true mastery requires diligence and dedication to moving the body and paying attention while doing so. It is the application of mindfulness to movement that enhances your Body Mind Intelligence.

Chapter Eight

Three Cheers for Body Mind Intelligence

I just remembered a cheer we did in junior high school. It went like this:

Lean to the left, lean to the right. Stand up, sit down. Fight fight fight!"

How funny is that? And the whole crowd would lean one way and then the other and stand up and sit down and yell. Sometimes we would go faster and faster until we couldn't keep up the motion. And we would laugh and laugh.

How often do you move just for the fun of it?

Do you ever wonder why you lost that spark of spontaneity for moving your body? And when did exercise replace our need to move?

The fact of the matter is, we were created for movement, not exercise. Yes, exercise is movement. But exercise can be nothing more than rote repetition. Movement does not have to be exercise. Movement requires an active engagement of the mind, exercise not necessarily.

In my experience, I have observed how frequently people choose to distract themselves when they exercise. Notice how many people watch TV as they walk on the treadmill at the "health" club. Check out the widespread use of earphones by those who are actively working out.

You can either pay attention to what your body is doing, or you can distract yourself with audio-visual devices. Please ask yourself, is that distraction necessary for you? What is it about your exercise program that makes you want to disconnect from your body? Are you still living above the neck while working out?

When I teach an "exercise" class, I can see that there are students who simply "see and do." To see and do means that they simply watch what I do and then copy it. This is particularly the case in a group aerobics class. For example, if I wave to a friend who happens to be walking behind the class that I am facing, I have seen at least half of the students wave back at me, simply because I raised my palm and wiggled my fingers. I swear there have been times when I scratched my nose, and my class followed suit. I have always found that to be a troubling sign of disconnection. I've often wondered how it is so many become like little robots, just copying the movements rather than creating and feeling the movements.

I want to encourage you to actively participate in your exercise program. When you move your body, pay attention to how it feels and what is happening as you move. Are you able to find pleasure in moving the body or not?

Somewhere along the way, moving the body became unpleasant; otherwise, you would not be seeking a way to avoid it. Is it the activity itself you wish to avoid or is it something else? If you can't enjoy the activity, are you receiving the benefits you desire? If you aren't enjoying moving your body, what is the likelihood that you will move at all? Do you have to force yourself to move your body? What is the block?

As a child you found joy in moving your body. Play was important to you as a child. And as you played and explored, your little body grew stronger.

And then what happened when you went off to school? You were asked to sit still and pay attention. Recess, the part of your school day when you got to actually move and play, was such a reward that it was taken away when you didn't sit still and pay attention.

To this day, physical education is valued so little compared to academics that it, along with the arts, is the first to be cut back when money gets tight.

We know that children actually learn better when they move. Symptoms of attention-deficit hyperactivity disorder (ADHD) improve with physical activity. Physical activity improves executive function, and schools that incorporate physical activity into their students' curriculum have better academic outcomes. Even with this knowledge, physical education is not valued as much as performance scores on a year-end test.

We need to dig deep and figure out why physical education is so undervalued. If we dig deeply enough, we may even discover why we have to disconnect from our bodies as we force ourselves to exercise.

OK, so I've just had a small personal rant about physical education. I am serious about finding the answers to my questions. Why is mental capacity valued over physical capacity, when both are needed to thrive? Why do you value intellect more than physical fitness? Why are you in your head more than in your body?

To keep your mind sharp, you need to learn new information and apply your mental skills in a novel manner. To keep your body functioning well, you also need to learn and develop new skills. Exercise, in its rote repetition, challenges you so little that you have to create a distraction in order to keep your mind occupied while you do it. Is it me, or do you also see the irony here?

Exercise has become something you "have to" do or "should" do. When viewed from the lens of obligation, exercise is bound to lose its appeal. Finding a way to make exercise fun, enjoyable, and challenging can change your perception. Make it something you like and you're more likely to continue. I can't even begin to count the number of times I've said that exact thing only to see the suggestion fall on deaf ears and blank faces. It's a great suggestion, but personally, I haven't seen it become a great motivator.

For many people, the words "fun" and "exercise" cannot occur in the same sentence. If I've heard it once, I've heard it hundreds of times: "I hate exercise." I don't think I've ever heard someone say "I hate fun." And what could possibly be fun about doing something you hate?

Which begs the next question—why do people hate exercise so much? Is it the word itself that conjures up an image of torture? Is it the activity that is unpleasant or is it the feelings associated with the activity? I know I ask lots of questions. I've been asking them for years.

But what's really important is what is going on with you. Do you exercise? Do you find it pleasant or unpleasant? Do you look forward to moving your body and do you enjoy the sensation of moving your body? Do you seek out novel ways to move and challenge your body?

Are you present when you exercise or do you separate yourself out? Are you paying attention to your body as you move or are you somewhere else?

"Exercise" is an activity done without being fully engaged. Moving your body with your full attention and being fully present requires Body Mind Intelligence.

You were born with Body Mind Intelligence. You were born with the ability to move, and as you grew, you explored your movement potential. You knew joy in moving your body and learning new skills.

That joy is still present. It may be hiding beneath less pleasant emotions, but it is there. Finding the joy may require some sifting through and letting go of some of that old "stuff" that is keeping you from moving your body.

Here's a little something you can try right now. Go back, way back to when you were a kid. Think about what was fun to you. What kinds of games did you play and enjoy? Rather than wistfully regret the loss of your childhood, hold onto that joyous playful feeling.

Now let's do our cheer.

Actively participate, right where you are, right now.

Ready?! OK! Let's go!

Lean to the left, lean to the right.

Stand up, sit down. Fight, fight, fight!!!

Chapter Nine

"Fizzy-Cali" Fit

I'm a sucker for cute animated films, so when I mention King Julian, the royal pain-in-the-patootie lemur from the *Madagascar* movies, you'll just have to excuse my juvenile taste. However, if you recall, there's a prominent scene when he sings as he dances and struts about unabashedly: "I like to move it, move it." Perhaps you've seen it. And if not, it's fun, it's motivating, and it makes you want to dance. It's a "just can't help myself" kind of tune.

Like King Julian, our bodies were created for joyful movement. All you have to do is play a rhythmic dance beat and even a toddler will bounce up and down with a big smile. The more you move, it seems, the more your body responds with ease and enthusiasm. The more you move, the more joy there is to discover.

Take a moment to ponder your movement roots. When you think about it, you realize that early humans were forced to move about in order to find food. Your hunter and gatherer forebears did not have food readily available. In order to eat, they had to move. Food was the reward for a job well done.

In the modern world, you do not have to grow or gather your food. You no longer have to go out and hunt for meat. Moving your body is no longer necessary in order for you to survive, at least, not as far as food consumption is concerned.

Now the necessity of moving your body has somehow been relegated to the realm of "I know I should, but I don't have time." When you are full from a good meal, you pat yourself on the belly and say something along the lines of "gee, now I have to exercise."

Exercise has become your replacement for moving the body naturally. Instead of burning calories to find food, you currently think of burning calories to *counteract,* not contribute to, your eating habits. Such a dramatic shift in your mind set must be terribly confusing for your body.

Modern culture values exercise as a means of burning calories. The more calories you burn, the higher the value becomes. Such a value placed upon moving the body is completely counter-intuitive to your need to move.

I find it fascinating that there is a trend towards eating a "paleo" diet based upon foods that were available to our earliest ancestors. Eating paleo is believed to be healthy because it is a diet that was intended to nourish the body when humans were hunting and gathering.

You want your foods to be organic, with no added pesticides or chemicals. You avoid genetically modified organism (GMOs) because you want your food to be in its natural state.

You realize that overly processed foods contribute to a diet that is lacking nutrients.

Yet, when it comes to moving your body, you exercise in a very un-paleo, un-organic manner. There is nothing natural about walking on a treadmill or pedaling the elliptical. Lifting weights is an artificial means of creating a workload that really does not resemble how the body moves in a real-life situation at all.

Just like food is nourishment for your body, so is movement. Good nutrition requires a variety of foods in order to meet your nutritional needs. Physical fitness requires a variety of ways of moving your body. The body requires movement just like it requires food.

Do you enjoy eating a variety of foods? Do you only eat broccoli? Of course you eat a variety of foods because you like them and because you know that your body needs nutrients from a variety of food sources. Think of movement exactly the same way—vary the activity, vary the motion.

Start an "organic" trend in moving your body. Begin by examining your common day-to-day activities, or lack thereof.

In what activities do you expend the most energy? When do you expend the least amount of energy? Do you spend more time moving or not moving?

Do you work in an office where you spend a lot of time sitting? Do you have a long commute sitting in the car or on the train? Do you work in a retail store where you spend a lot of your time standing?

I used to believe that exercise could counteract the effects of sitting. Recently, I have seen some convincing studies that indicate the risks of sitting cannot be overcome even with regular exercise. The most recent study was published in the *Annals of Internal Medicine* in January 2015. Conducted by Aviroop Biswas and colleagues, this systemic review and meta-analysis showed that sitting contributes to the development of cardiovascular disease, cancer, and type II diabetes, independent of exercise. The hazards of sitting were less pronounced in those who reported more activity than those who remained sedentary, but it could not eliminate the risk.

If the risks of sitting are so great and exercise cannot necessarily counter the effect, what is one to do? Start moving more. Sit less.

As stated earlier, exercise is movement, but movement is not necessarily exercise. Incorporating movement regularly into your routine can have a tremendous impact on your health and well-being.

There is no set amount or threshold to try to achieve. Simply find ways to move. If you sit, stand up every 10–15 minutes or try to move about for a few minutes every hour. Don't just sit and sit and sit. Move, fidget, stand up, and dance. Whatever you choose to do, just move more.

If you simply stood up from your seat once every 15 minutes and took 3 minutes per hour to move, at the end of the day, you have accumulated about 45 minutes of moving into your day. I would call that a very good start!

Why not turn finding ways to move into a little game you play? Make it fun whatever you do. No need to turn moving your body into another "should."

Be aware of not moving and change it slightly. Sitting still with crossed legs? Wiggle your foot. Uncross and stretch and cross the other way. Stand up and readjust. Don't just sit there—move something!

Here's a little something I discovered that helps me incorporate balance and flexibility moves into my day. When I get dressed, I avoid sitting down. I put on my clothes, including shoes and socks, from a standing position. Maybe it doesn't seem like much, but give it a try tomorrow morning when you are getting dressed for the day. See what kind of challenges it presents for you.

How are you with getting up and down from the floor? That's a movement challenge that many people have. And your ability to move up and down from the floor has been shown to predict longevity. In a study published in the *European Journal of Preventive Cardiology* in December

2012, researchers from Brazil used a sitting-rising test (SRT) and discovered that those who scored well and could easily sit and rise from the floor without assistance lived longer and were less likely to die from any given cause than those who had difficulty with sitting and rising. This simple musculoskeletal fitness test does a remarkable job of predicting longevity and gives you even more reason to keep moving and improving what your body can do.

In addition to living longer, being physically active also increases your chances of living independently and enjoying a greater quality of life. Quite frankly, living long really is not as important as living well and being able to maintain the activities of daily living. I believe we all seek to live an independent and active lifestyle. Living well has far more value than living long.

So what do you need to do to continue to live well? Move your body. A sedentary lifestyle results in loss of muscle mass, loss of bone density, diminished aerobic capacity, poor posture, and increased fatigability. If you want to maintain your balance, your strength, your coordination, and your stamina, choose to move.

Now that you are making an effort to incorporate a variety of moves into your activities of daily living, let's examine what kind of moves you already have in your daily repertoire. If you exercise regularly, good for you! Exercise is important and vital to your health and well-being. You already know the benefits!

The wider the variety of movements and the frequency with which you move makes a difference as well. Keep in mind that although exercise is movement, it may not provide an adequate variety of movement to give you a well-balanced fitness program.

I have always taught that a well-balanced fitness program has cardiorespiratory, strength, and flexibility components. It is important to do your cardio. It is important to lift weights and stretch. Of course I am going to encourage you to try and incorporate each of these elements into your fitness routines. However, I now realize that it is vitally important to avoid sitting for long periods of time; therefore, moving intermittently throughout the day contributes significantly to your physical fitness and capacity. It also helps you avoid the risks and losses that accompany not moving.

Obviously, for your benefit, a balance must be struck. It is possible to move too much, that is, more than your body can handle at any one time or over an extended time period. How do you discover what is appropriate for you?

I encourage you to consider how to achieve variety in your movement plan to keep your body fit, healthy, and injury-free. Repeating the same motion over and over again, although it challenges your cardiorespiratory system, may be taxing your musculoskeletal system through repetitive motion. The primary cause of injury in any exercise program is overuse. Learning your body's tolerance level and capacity for moving is going to demand your attention. You have to take responsibility for learning your body's limitations and potential.

I can't begin to tell you how many clients I have worked with who stopped their previous exercise programs because of injury. How about you? Have you ever experienced an overuse injury as a result of exceeding your personal limitations? Is there any chance that what you are doing for exercise right now could possibly be injuring you at the same time?

Don't let your exercise program be the cause of you not moving your body. Seek a variety of movement in your exercise plan as well as in your activities of daily living, and you will feel better as a result.

Now consider your day-to-day environment. What keeps you sitting still and what keeps you moving? Thanks to modern technology, you don't even have to get up to answer the phone or change stations on the television. When was the last time you rolled down a car window or dialed a telephone?

All these small changes in your physical environment save you time and energy, but they also prevent you from moving your body with the frequency and variety you need.

Technology is wonderful in how it has expanded your connection with the world. But what about your connection with the self, with your body? Can you think of ways that technology keeps you from moving your body? Does a computer keep you sitting at your desk?

Amazing how something so good for you can be your own undoing. So, in order to counter the hazardous effect of sitting, the "cure" is greater frequency of movement rather than increased amount or intensity. Set a goal of moving once every 10–15 minutes when sitting. Walk across the room and back. Stand on one leg. Raise your arms and stretch.

Have fun with it.

Make a game of it.

It's not work when you're just trying to be "fizzy-cali fit."

Chapter Ten

Physically Fit

How do you measure health? Think about it. Is optimal health the absence of disease or the presence of vitality? What is the difference between being well and being ill?

Doctors use a variety of measures to determine how the body functions to decide if you need treatment or not. Using the best methods available to them, they look to see what illnesses or problems exist. Simple measurements such as blood pressure or temperature give information to let your doctor know whether something is amiss. If your temperature is high, an infection is likely present. In that case, another test may be performed to discover the type of infection so that you receive the appropriate treatment. Accurate diagnostic testing leads to appropriate treatments.

Blood pressure and pulse measurements are used as indicators of cardiovascular health. If additional information is indicated, an electrocardiogram (EKG) gives a little closer look at how the heart is functioning and helps ascertain if there are any problems with cardiac rhythm or conductivity. For an even closer look, there are multiple tests that can be used to investigate the heart's function. From echocardiograms to catheterizations, tests become more sophisticated and specialized depending on the information necessary for your doctor to determine the best method of treatment for your particular situation or problem.

As complex and sophisticated as medical testing has become, using body weight alone as a measure of health seems rather antiquated and primitive. Therefore, the recommendation of weight loss based simply upon stepping on a scale and determining that your BMI does not fall within the recommended range makes very little sense. More sophisticated testing would be necessary to determine if there was an underlying medical issue, and there is no reasonable need to treat weight in the absence of any problems or symptoms.

The mere absence of symptoms, however, is not the equivalent or determinant of optimal health. Health and vitality are associated with being physically fit, and physical fitness is closely related to positive health outcomes. It seems obvious that we should place more emphasis on the assessment of fitness and not on BMI.

The use of Vimdex helps us to self-assess as we begin to manage our personal energy more effectively. However, if medicine and science need an objective measure as well in order to determine the efficacy of any intervention, then what reasonable or accurate measure exists?

Vimdex, as a self-assessment tool, gives us great personal health and vitality information but is not scientifically valid until it is used and compared with health-related outcomes. In short, more data are needed. Fortunately, for science's sake, we do have methods available to us that are able to accurately reflect changes in the human body relative to the influence of physical activity.

The health-related *measurable* components of physical fitness are as follows: (1) cardiorespiratory endurance, (2) muscular endurance, (3) muscular strength, (4) body composition, and (5) flexibility. As an exercise physiologist, much of my own education and training focused upon how to assess and improve each of these components of fitness as it relates to health.

Physical fitness has been defined by the President's Council on Physical Fitness and Sports as "the ability to carry out daily tasks with vigor and alertness, without undue fatigue and with ample energy to enjoy leisure-time pursuits and to meet unforeseen emergencies." Other definitions include "a state of well-being with low risk of premature health problems and energy to participate in a variety of physical activities" (Howley and Franks, 1997). It is apparent that even by these definitions, terms such as vigor, alertness, fatigue, and energy are difficult to measure.

To help you determine how to measure your personal energy levels, I have introduced Vimdex as an expression of vim, vigor, and vitality. Perhaps one day, Vimdex will be an accepted measure of energy in the scientific community, but until then, it can certainly help you keep track of how you are feeling on a day-to-day basis. For now, feel free to use Vimdex as it pleases you.

We do have the ability to measure the health-related attributes of physical fitness in a very scientific manner. Cardiorespiratory endurance (aerobic capacity) is expressed in terms of oxygen uptake, how well the body is able to put oxygen to use in order to provide the energy necessary to perform any given task. Typical testing methods include treadmill or cycling tests, in which oxygen uptake is measured through a breathing apparatus or estimated based upon the workload achieved.

There are a variety of methods to test muscular strength and flexibility. Grip strength is frequently used as a measure of muscular strength. The sit-and-reach test is often employed as a measure of hip flexibility. Although these tests are rather specific, they are frequently utilized to express relative strength and flexibility.

The measurement and evaluation of each of the components of fitness have value as you pursue the enjoyment of your physical health. As your physical capacity improves, you will observe measurable differences in your aerobic capacity, endurance, strength, and flexibility.

The health-related components of physical fitness improve even in the absence of weight loss. Therefore, health benefits may be gained from the pursuit of physical fitness without any change in body weight.

It is critical to note that it is body composition—not body weight—that comprises one of the primary components of physical fitness. Body composition relates to the relative amounts of muscle, fat, bone, and organs that make up the vital parts of the body. As muscle tissue and bone mass contribute to the ability to remain physically active, we must address any loss of muscle or bone mass as a serious health risk.

Proponents of physical fitness often refer to the fact that muscle mass is more metabolically active and burns more calories than fat mass. We also hear that muscle weighs more than fat. Logic tells us that is essentially wrong, as five pounds of fat weighs exactly the same as five pounds of muscle. The true difference is volume and density. Muscle mass is more dense and takes up less space than fat mass.

Since half of our body mass is skeletal muscle tissue, which is essential to movement and metabolism, any loss may have an extremely negative impact on health and well-being. A health concern related to dieting with the sole purpose of weight loss is the loss of lean muscle mass along with the loss of fat mass. In addition to decreased mobility and function, loss of muscle also results in increased fatigue and risk of metabolic disorders such as diabetes.

Body composition, as a health-related component of physical fitness, has been measured historically through various methods such as underwater weighing, bio electrical impedance, air displacement plethysmography, and skinfolds. Today's most modern, widely accepted test for body composition is dual-energy X-ray absorptiometry, or DEXA. DEXA is also more frequently utilized in the measurement of bone density, but body density can be accurately measured as well and with relative ease.

Body mass index was at first thought to be closely related to body composition, but it does not and cannot accurately reflect the internal makeup of the human body. It is possible to have a BMI considered to be healthy that, in reality, may be extremely unhealthy because of low muscle and bone mass. Measuring body composition can help assess the relative amount of fat and lean tissue in the body and serves as a more accurate reflection of the impact of physical activity on the metabolic profile.

Body composition measurements are expressed as body fat percentage or the amount of fat present relative to total body mass. While there remains some association between body fat percentage and health, where your fat tends to be stored appears to be the higher risk associated with the development of cardiovascular disease.

Abdominal fat content can be accurately measured with radiological imaging techniques such as DEXA and magnetic resonance imaging (MRI). Waist circumference measurement may be utilized as a simpler test to reflect abdominal fat storage and is associated with cardiometabolic disease risk.

The greater association remains between cardiorespiratory fitness measures and health outcomes. Since aerobic exercise has been shown to reduce both waist circumference and cardiometabolic risk in the absence of weight loss, it appears, once again, that the most important factor in influencing health outcomes related to body fat is the practice of moving the body.

In summary, the health-related components of physical fitness are measurable. As fitness improves, you have more energy, but we do not yet possess a scientific measure of that feeling. You may choose to measure the attributes of physical fitness in order to measure your personal progress. Or you may choose to use Vimdex as a personal expression of how great it feels to be physically fit.

Chapter Eleven

Quiet the Riot

Please understand that the energy you have to give at any given moment of the day is directly related to what you think and how you move. Your vitality is a balance achieved between moving your body and quieting your mind.

At this point, you have just learned that small, frequent, intermittent, and varied doses of physical activity help to keep your body functioning optimally. Moving your body prevents the loss of strength and stamina that results from a sedentary lifestyle. Moving your body prepares and fortifies your body for what you may ask it to do for you at any given time, helping you manage your very busy life.

Rumination of the mind and stagnation of the body are draining to your energy stores. To restore your energy balance, move your body and quiet your mind—the foundation of Body Mind Intelligence.

The practice of mindfulness allows you to become aware of the thoughts that may be draining your energy or having a negative impact on your body. Runaway thoughts of worry and anxiety take your energy away because of the energy required to maintain those negative thoughts.

Practicing mindfulness does not mean you stop thinking; instead, you are aware of the thoughts and become an observer of them in order to diminish the emotional charge that you attach to them. The practice of mindfulness is often thought to be the act of meditation. Although it is a meditative practice, it can be applied to any activity or circumstance.

Mindfulness helps improve your resilience, your ability to recover from and deal with negative events. Mindfulness practice also reduces your physiological stress response. You become less reactive; therefore, your body sustains less of a hit from your emotions.

A pioneer in the field of mindfulness meditation, Jon Kabat-Zinn defines mindfulness as "paying attention on purpose, in the present moment and without judgment." It is a way of living and being.

As you become better at observing and not judging your thoughts, you cultivate greater compassion for yourself as well as others. Compassion for self is a vital component of Body Mind Intelligence. Rather than beating yourself up for gaining weight, far better to accept what is and move on with a loving and positive approach towards your body. Give yourself a whole lotta love.

Mindfulness means living in the moment and being fully aware of all that is happening right in front of you. Being mindful is being present with both your mind and your body. In practicing mindfulness, you notice and pay attention to the sensations and feelings that arise in your body as part of being present and fully aware. Being mindful, despite the way it sounds, is about getting out of your head and into your body.

Practicing mindfulness means paying attention to your body and feelings. In mindfulness meditation, you notice your body and your feelings. A meditative practice asks you to become the observer of your body in addition to your thoughts. Sometimes the practice of sitting still in meditation is difficult because of those feelings that inevitably arise. Being able to sit with your feelings, without judgment, is a challenge. That is why it takes a great deal of practice to get better at observing and being present.

Mindfulness meditation does not require a trance-like, empty mind. Instead, it requires stillness and discipline to just be with your thoughts and feelings, something that many of us find excruciating. I encourage you to try mindfulness meditation and become more tolerant of those uncomfortable, uneasy feelings.

If you find sitting still to be too difficult, it is possible to put mindfulness into practice in other ways. Body Mind Intelligence encourages a mindful approach to moving your body, paying attention to the feelings and sensations in your body as you move, rather than just sitting still. Sitting in stillness and mindfully moving your body can both benefit your body and your sense of well-being.

Combining the concept of mindfulness with moving the body is the practice of yoga, which has been used as "exercise" for millennia. Intended as a means to prepare the body for meditation, yoga impacts the flow of energy through the body. In yoga, it is believed that energy can get stuck in the body because of injury or trauma, whether physical or emotional. By moving the body through the performance of certain asanas or poses, this block can be released.

The purpose of each asana is to allow the flow of energy through the body, represented by the seven chakras or energy centers. Ranging in location from the base of the spinal column through the crown of the head, the chakras hold a connection to the divine. If energy can flow through the body, represented by the chakras, the channel to the divine remains open and clear.

Anapanasati is a form of Buddhist meditation, but it is now utilized in Western-based mindfulness practices. "Anapana" means inhalation and exhalation, and "sati" refers to mindfulness. Anapanasati means to feel the sensations in the body caused by the breath.

The use of the breath is emphasized in yoga and is the starting point for nearly all meditative practices. Mindfulness meditation uses anapanasati as a focus during the meditation. Pranayama, or breath control, is taught in both traditional and modern forms of yoga. The breath is used as a focal point in connecting with your body. Your ability to connect with your body through the breath is a foundational practice of Body Mind Intelligence.

Chapter Twelve

Creating Balance: The Power of Not Doing

I spent years focusing on "doing" the exercise and then I made a breakthrough discovery: the importance of rest. It is so easy to focus on the action of movement so much that you lose sight of the second half of the fitness equation. To improve your physical capacity, you need to achieve a balance of work *and* rest.

Work can be defined as the stimulus necessary to create a demand on the body. Rest is allowing the body the time to adapt to the demand.

Weight-lifting recovery time is a great example of the importance of rest. First, the weight creates the workload that places a demand on the body, all the way down to the level of the muscle cell. The demand actually causes disruption and damage at the cellular level. In order for the body to accommodate the workload the next time you go to the gym and lift that same weight, it has to heal and become more resilient to the demand. That time of healing and strengthening requires, on average, around 48 hours. That is why you have most likely been instructed to lift weights on nonconsecutive days.

Of course, sleep is the quintessential example of resting your body. You know that sleep is important to your health.

It is the period of time that your body recovers and rests so that you can continue to do things (perform in life) the next day. Without sleep, your body cannot function optimally. Yet, it is the first thing that gets sacrificed in order to meet the demands of daily living.

In case you haven't noticed, you live in a land of the sleep deprived. There are zombies all around you, operating on too little sleep and putting their health, and yours, at risk as a result. What about you? Can you count yourself among the walking dead? Chances are at some point, you have experienced the zombie state. We all have.

Placing demands on the body without allowing adequate time for rest and recovery leads to further degradation and disruption. Eventually, it fails. Sound familiar to you?

Have you ever put yourself in a situation where you felt that you exceeded what your body could handle either intentionally or unintentionally? For example, have you ever stayed up late night after night in order to meet a deadline? You finished the project (hooray for you!) and then you came down with a cold—or worse.

Your body needs you to rest just as much as it needs you to work. Both have value! And one is not more valuable than the other, even though we are led to believe that what we are "doing" is way more important than what we are "not doing." This is sometimes called "work-life" balance.

Fascinating, because that statement makes it sound like there's work and then everything else is your life. Doesn't it seem that there is no such thing as work-life balance since most often it is your "work," what you "do," that is what defines you?

When people ask what you do, what do you say? Do you tell them you go to bed and sleep 8 hours every night? Do you tell them that you move your body in magnificent ways every day? Or do you tell them what you do for work?

If you live in the United States, you also live in a vacation-deprived nation. We live in the only nation amongst the world's major economies that does not mandate vacation time or sick time. Perhaps the remainder of the modern world sees the value in allowing the body to take time to rest and recover. The United States apparently sees more value in working your body to death—literally!

You can never be "rich enough or thin enough." Being rich enough requires you to work, work, work, and that will make you sick. Being thin enough means you will be constantly unhappy with your body, and that will make you sick.

And on top of it all, your health is not necessarily your right but a commodity that makes money for an industry that comprises 18% of the US gross domestic product. We should start calling it our "sick" care system, because it is not supporting our health and well-being.

Wake up from your zombie state and start paying attention to how often your health is viewed as a potential for profit. Notice how many pharmaceutical ads show you how you can feel better if you would just get your doctor to prescribe this particular medicine for you. Notice how many ads you see for hip and knee replacements. Contrast that with any ads that encourage you to be physically active or practice mindfulness.

Health care in the United States is the most expensive in the world, yet it ranks low in terms of quality. According to *Time* magazine's June 17, 2014 issue, "The U.S. ranks worst among 11 wealthy nations in terms of 'efficiency, equity and outcomes' despite having the world's most expensive health care system."

There are a chorus of complaints about Obamacare and the costs; however, keep in mind that the health care (ahem, "sick" care) system that has been in place for years contributes to the high costs, not just what has happened since the implementation of the Affordable Care Act. Have you heard the health insurance companies complaining recently?

So if you do not want, or cannot expect, government involvement in your healthcare, you must take direct responsibility for your own body and your own health.

That begins with adequate rest, proper nutrition, moving the body, and quieting the mind.

No one else is going to do it for you.

You believe you need to be rich and thin. And where did you get the idea that you cannot be thin enough or rich enough? It has been brilliantly marketed to you because as long as you fear you are not enough or don't possess enough, you are willing to spend your hard-earned money to get what you need.

You are bombarded with messages every single day, carefully crafted for your money. Capitalism provides you the opportunity to be as rich or as thin as you would like, but there is a price to be paid. That price is your money and your health.

Your money follows your values. Watch where it goes. Who receives most of your money and why?

Your energy follows your money. Watch where it goes. Where do you expend the greatest amount of your energy and why? Is your health being sacrificed in that pursuit?

Creating the balance between work and rest is critical to your health and well-being. If there is no other point to be made in your understanding of Body Mind Intelligence, it is this one truth: your beliefs are reflected in your body. When you choose to sacrifice the health needs of your body in your pursuit of something else, your body suffers. When you choose to appreciate and care for your body, it flourishes and thrives.

Do you prefer to survive or thrive?

You have to determine where your own values lie and where you "have to" put your energy. Are you focusing on your health or your wealth? Are you focusing on your well-being or on the scale? Are you rich enough or thin enough?

As long as you believe you are not enough, you suffer. And your body will reflect your feelings of inadequacy. Your negative thoughts of not being enough or not having enough will show up in your body, in one way or another. But know this truth as well: your health depends upon your belief that you are enough and you have enough. Too often you feel that you live in lack. Your feelings of lack contribute to lack of energy, lack of vitality, and lack of enthusiasm. Your body suffers.

Are you thinking to yourself, "But if I were rich and thin, I would be happy"? Why would that make you happy? I'm certain it would not be a surprise to you to learn that being thin and being rich does not equate to happiness.

To feel better and to have more energy is going to require a shift in your thoughts and beliefs. You must believe that your body deserves appreciation and gratitude for providing a way for you to exist in this world. Take a moment to reflect upon this gift. You were born with the body you have; it is yours to appreciate and provide the care it needs.

Self-care is your responsibility. Your body and your health are your responsibility, *not your health care provider's.*

When you feel sick, your doctor prescribes a treatment for your symptoms. Your illness is a manifestation of a systemic problem. You are far more capable of determining the root cause of your illness than your doctor. Your doctor treats symptoms and diseases. Being well requires your attention. It's your body and your relationship with your body that ultimately matters.

If your health is suffering or you don't have the energy you need to complete the tasks of everyday life, you may have some serious self-examination to do. Perhaps someone else's needs are being put before your own. Perhaps it is a complete disconnect from your body and your own inability to respond to its needs.

If you are not taking full responsibility for your well-being, someone else will. If you do not determine your own set of values, there are plenty of people who will tell you what your values should be and where you should be spending your time and money.

Self-care is not a selfish act. Your life depends upon it.

Is your life a reflection of what you really want? Do you believe that in order for you to have the money you need that you cannot "afford" to take care of your own body? Do you operate from the belief that you can never be rich enough?

Health and wealth are not thin and rich.

All too often, it is your health that suffers as you continue to operate from the belief that you cannot be too rich or too thin. What weight is thin enough for you? How much money is rich enough for you? Both are unattainable goals because they don't exist. The *truth* is you *cannot* be too rich or too thin.

In your pursuit of rich enough or thin enough, are you willing to stop and take a good long look at your values. Jesus himself asked, "What does it profit a man to gain the whole world but to lose his own soul?" Are you willing to open your eyes to see where your life is out of balance?

I encourage you to take out a sheet of paper and draw 2 columns.

Resources

Money	Time

Now write down how you allocate these resources in your life. Where you choose to spend your time and your money are a direct reflection of your personal values and your beliefs.

How much of your time is allocated for rest or sleep?

How much time do you spend sitting over the course of the day?

How much time do you spend in the car sitting and driving?

How is your money allocated?

How much time do you spend worrying?

How much time do you worry about money?

How much of your time is used towards meeting someone else's goals?

How much time and/or money is allocated to your personal well-being?

Are you satisfied with the distribution of your resources?

Are there imbalances anywhere?

Consider that time is money and money is energy.

The allocation of your time and money is the perfect representation of your energy expenditure.

Your energy is your body's resource that it needs to perform the activities of your day-to-day life. If your body's energy stores are depleted, it cannot provide you the support and assistance you may be requiring of it on a day-to-day basis. The more energy required by your life, the less vitality your body has to offer, unless you are willing to allocate the resources of time and money to take care of you.

Your energy goes where you intend it to go, based upon your value system.

What do you think is easier to do: allocate your resources differently or change your value system?

Body Mind Intelligence requires that you know exactly where your values lie and live your life accordingly. If thin and rich are important to you, it is your privilege to pursue them, but you do so now with the knowledge that thin and rich are elusive and unattainable, as well as an enormous drain of your precious resources.

If you value your health, your relationship with your body becomes a vital part of your value system. When you value your relationship with your body, you discover how your allocation of resources shifts and changes. When you value your relationship with your body, you are willing to stop and rest because you either anticipated the needs of your body or you are listening when the body says "enough."

Your body needs you to believe that you are enough. Your body needs you to be present more than it needs you to "do" anything.

When you value your relationship with your body, you show your appreciation by providing it with the care and attention it deserves. And you are willing to allocate time and money (your energy) to maintain and cultivate that relationship.

Perhaps the greatest gift you can give to yourself is to honor your physical self. Your body requires your love, attention, support, and care.

How have you expressed your gratitude for your body today?

What can you "not do" to your body to say thank you?

Chapter Thirteen

A Matter of Trust

Cultivating and enhancing your relationship with your body enables you to tap into your body's wisdom. A level of trust is established between you and your body so that you feel that the body is more responsive to what you need. You are able to trust the messages and feelings from your body and the information that your body provides for you.

That trust in the body is developed through cultivating the relationship with the body. How easy is it for you to translate wanting to create a certain movement with the body and your body's ability to perform that specific movement? Any physical skill is going to require a conversation between you and your body. Typically, the more open the lines of communication are, the higher the skill level becomes.

Athletes and dancers demonstrate their relationship with their bodies through their performances. They are able to move without thinking "how" to make it happen. When a level of performance is achieved and it seems effortless, that is mastery. That kind of response from the body is the result of time spent in training and in relationship with the body.

Athletes care for their bodies, getting just the right amount of rest and nutrition the body needs to perform optimally. A trust relationship is established. A great performance is far more likely to result from a trusting relationship between the athlete and her body when trust is present and the body's needs are being met.

An athlete understands that you don't pull a series of all-nighters to prepare your body for an Olympic competition. An athlete knows that you don't go to the vending machine for a nourishing meal. An athlete has spent years developing skills and is going to make sure that the body gets what it needs to perform at the highest level possible.

You may not be a professional athlete who depends on the optimal performance of the body, but if you seek optimal health, you must develop the same appreciation for what the body does and needs. You must develop the same relationship of trust. When you act as if your body will take care of itself and ignore its needs, the relationship suffers and your health suffers.

I have purposefully not addressed nutrition and food in this discussion of Body Mind Intelligence. That is not because I don't believe that good nutrition is important. It is because that is not my area of expertise or what I feel is within my scope of practice. Furthermore, it has always been my experience that plenty of great nutrition information is readily available. Most of my clients already have a good working knowledge of nutrition. The confusion occurs with all the noise from the diet industry that clamors for their attention.

I have also discovered that once the conversation around food begins, that becomes the focal point. It is as if there is nothing else that can be done. The diet industry has done a perfect job of convincing you that food is the determining factor for everything related to the body and health. While there is an element of truth there, factors other than what you eat work together to create health and well-being. This entire book has focused upon your relationship with your body. Looking for someone to tell you what to eat is a perfect example of being disconnected from your body.

Eat what you determine is proper nutrition for you. Don't let the diet industry tell you. You have to determine what your body needs and how to provide it. If you really don't know what foods are best for you, please seek the advice of a dietitian.

It is disheartening to witness how many people become so caught up in "food rules." From my point of view, the more rules that exist around your food, the more disordered your eating becomes. While having food rules may not mean you have an eating disorder, it is exhibiting an unhealthy relationship with food.

A healthy relationship with food indicates a healthy relationship with the body. I would even be tempted to say that the more disconnected the relationship is with your body, the more likely you are to exhibit disordered eating patterns.

If you find that you are overly preoccupied with food or overly concerned about your appearance, you may be at risk for an eating disorder. If you feel you cannot trust yourself around food or you experience guilt in relation to eating, you may be at risk for an eating disorder.

I cannot, in good conscience, complete this book without mentioning eating disorders. It is a serious medical condition that requires professional help. It is not in the scope of this book to treat an eating disorder, therefore I feel it is my obligation to make my audience aware that they themselves may be suffering from or at risk of developing an eating disorder such as anorexia nervosa, bulimia, or binge eating disorder. The following organizations have information online, and I recommend a visit to their websites: the National Eating Disorder Association, Multi-Service Eating Disorder Association, and Binge Eating Disorder Association.

You may have noticed that I have stayed away from any exercise "rules" as well. It is my personal philosophy that first we must establish a healthy relationship with the body rather than meet the recommended requirements for exercise.

I consider counting calories to be counter to the philosophy of cultivating a healthy relationship with the body. It places a value on the food or on the exercise that relates more to body size than it does to your health. Counting calories may serve its purpose in demonstrating the caloric density or nutritional content of a food, but it does not make it "good" or "bad." The same is true for exercise. Just because a particular activity burns more calories does not make it a better choice.

Placing the labels of good and bad onto a food is placing a moral judgment for which, quite frankly, the food cannot be held responsible. It is your perception of the good or bad that makes it what it is. And it is your perception of the food that makes the difference in how your body responds. Remember the indulgent shake we discussed earlier? The *belief* that it provided more calories was enough to convince the body it was satisfied. What do you think might happen in your body when you call the food you just consumed bad for you?

The body reflects your beliefs in your health and your vitality.

Your primary concern is cultivating a healthy relationship with your body. From my experience and from scientific research, I have come to this conclusion. Two of the best behaviors you can adopt that can make the biggest change in your overall health are these: (1) move the body and (2) quiet the mind.

Both physical activity and mindfulness have proven to be quite effective in eliciting positive healthy responses in the body, even down to the ability to change your DNA at the cellular level. Your Body Mind Intelligence reflects your relationship with your body. When you initiate moving the body, paying attention to the body's response establishes a line of communication and trust.

As the body accommodates and adapts to you asking it to move, it becomes even more resilient and capable. As you become more aware of the body and aware of your feelings, you become more resilient and capable. A relationship of mutual trust follows.

Your intellect cannot act without the body. Your intelligence manifests in your ability to relate to and with your body. As you grow in your appreciation of your body and as you learn to care for its needs, you will flourish and thrive.

Thrive in your newly discovered relationship. Get out of your head and into your heart and soul.

Discover your Body Mind Intelligence.

Chapter 14

Dance to the Rhythm of Life

You and your body are now engaged in conversation. This ongoing dialogue results in you feeling better and having more energy. You ask the body to move, and it responds.

Your body has the remarkable capacity to adapt and respond to the demands of physical activity. Yet, sometimes it cannot, and injury results. Your conversation continues as you must now focus on the healing process. Your body's capacity to heal is directly related to your willingness to pay attention to what the body needs in this process.

You have to learn the dance of asking and receiving so that your body can heal and adapt. If you remain present, you and your body dance together beautifully. If you choose to not listen, the dance is over. If you fail to ask, the dance can never even begin.

Learning to dance requires discipline, partnership, and trust. Being in the dance has its challenges and its rewards, and it is up to you how dedicated and involved you are in this partnership and process—you and your body and your dance.

Your dance is unique, shaped by your partnership and your history, all viewed through your eyes, your lens. You have a different lens and a story all your own. The choices you make for your body will not be the same as the choices I make for mine. My dance is all my own, viewed through a different lens.

You determine what needs to be addressed in order for you to have the enthusiasm and vitality you need to live your life. You know better than anyone where your energy goes and you must begin to manage it well.

With Body Mind Intelligence, you learn to focus your lens as you learn to manage also your output of energy both physically and emotionally. Being connected to your body allows you the privilege of recognizing feelings and responding as you choose. This is part of the dance.

You become far less likely to give your energy away by allowing circumstances or people you cannot control to have power over you. Body Mind Intelligence is the knowledge that feelings are information from your body. Having that knowledge allows you to respond with reason. Having emotions is to be fully human.

Body Mind Intelligence allows us to be human. It is what makes us human be-ings, not just humans do-ing. We have a choice, in being or in doing.

Moving your body is your choice. Paying attention to your body is your choice. Your health and your vitality—also your choice.

We realize that there are illnesses and diseases we do not choose for ourselves. We also agree that our response to sickness impacts our health outcomes. If you believe that stress will make you sick, it most likely will. If you believe that you and your body can work together, you can heal.

If you believe that your well-being is threatened and you are afraid, your body reacts to your fears. If you choose to realize that stress is created from your perceptions and you choose to perceive differently, it loses its power over you. Your body does not have to expend energy to address the threat. You have the power to determine your own course of action, your own interpretation of the dance.

Your dance is about connection. As you learn to connect with your body, your Body Mind Intelligence grows. You become increasingly more responsive to your body and what it has to say. As you become more connected to your body, you enhance your ability to discern what really requires your attention and focus and what does not.

With the dance, you develop a sense of trust and understanding. Your relationship with your body deepens so that you become better at recognizing and responding to the messages your body holds for you. You can trust the wisdom of the body. It is the chatter of the mind that breaks the connection.

It is a dance of energy. You cannot see it, but you can certainly feel it. When you dance with your body with the intention of love and care, you discover how your body responds by having more energy available for you.

Your path to health begins with your own awareness and is sustained through appreciation and care for your physical self.

You are growing and expanding in Body Mind Intelligence. The more you dance, the more you will know. The more you know, the better you will feel.

A New BMI will lead you down your path to better health and enhanced well-being.

You are dancing to the rhythm of life.

Enjoy the dance.

References and Recommended Reading

Chapter One:

Barry VW, Baruth M, Beets MW, Durstine JL, Lin J, Blair SN. Fitness vs. fatness on all-cause mortality: a meta-analysis. *Prog Cardiovasc Dis.* 2014 Jan-Feb; 56(4): 382-390.

Blair SN, Kohl HW 3rd, Barlow CE, Paffenbarger RS Jr, Gibbons CW, Maccra CA. Changes in physical fitness and all cause mortality. A prospective study of healthy and unhealthy men. *JAMA.* 1995 Apr 12; 273(14): 1093-1098.

Blair SN, Kohl HW 3rd, Paffenbarger RS Jr, Clark DG, Cooper KH, Gibbons LW. Physical fitness and all-cause mortality. A prospective study of healthy men and women. *JAMA.* 1989 Nov 3; 262(17): 2395-2401.

Fildes A, Charlton J, Rudisill C, Littlejohns P, Prevost AT, Gulliford MC. Probability of an obese person attaining normal body weight: cohort study using electronic health records. *Am J Public Health.* 2015 July 16. doi: 10.2105/AJPH.2015.302773

Flegal KM, Fit BK, Orpana H, Graubard BI. Association of all-cause mortality with overweight and obesity using standard body mass index categories: a systematic review and meta-analysis. *JAMA.* 2013 Jan 2; 309(1): 71-82.

Chapter Two:

Myss, C. *Anatomy of the Spirit.* New York: Harmony Books; 1996. pp. 40-43.

Chapter Three:
Bowman, K. *Move Your DNA: Restore Your Health Through Natural Movement.* Carlsborg, WA: Propriometrics Press; 2014. pp. 64-73.

Hart LE. Exercise and soft tissue injury. *Baillieres Clin Rheumatol.* 1994 Feb; 8(1): 137-148.

O'Keefe JH, Vogel R, Lavie CJ, Cordain L. Achieving hunter-gatherer fitness in the 21st century: back to the future. *Am J Med.* 2010 Dec; 123(12): 1082-1086.

Chapter Four:
Bacon L, Aphramor L. Weight science: evaluating the evidence for a paradigm shift. *Nutr J.* 2011 Jan; 10:9.

Puhl RM, Latner JD, O'Brien K, Luedicke J, Forhan M, Danielsdottir S. Cross national perspectives about weight based bullying in youth: nature, extent and remedies. *Pediatr Obes.* 2015 July 6. doi: 10.1111/ijpo.12051.

Puhl RM, Heuer CA. Obesity stigma: important considerations for public health. *Am J Public Health.* 2010; 100(6): 1019-1028.

Puhl RM, Heuer CA. The stigma of obesity: a review and update. *Obesity* 2009 May; 17(5): 941-964.

Chapter Five:
Crum AJ, Corbin WR, Brownell KD. Mind over milkshakes: mindsets, not just nutrients, determine ghrelin response.

Health Psychol. 2011 Jul; 30(4): 424-429; discussion 430-431.

Chapter Six:
Vernikos J, Schneider V. Space, gravity and the physiology of aging: parallel or convergent disciplines? A mini-review. *Gerontology* 2010; 56(2): 157-166.

Vernikos, J. Sitting Kills, Moving Heals: How Simple Everyday Movement Will Prevent Pain, Illness, and Early Death – And Exercise Won't. Fresno, CA: Quill Driver Books; 2011.

Chapter Seven:
Farb N, Daubenmier J, Price C, et al. Interoception, contemplative practice, and health. *Front Psychol.* 2015 Jun 9; 6: 763.

Grecucci A, Pappaianni E, Siugzaite R, Theuninck A, Job R. Mindful emotion regulation: exploring the neurocognitive mechanisms behind mindfulness. *Biomed Res Int.* 2015 Jun 7; 2015: 670724.

Khoury B, Sharma M, Rush SE, Fournier C. Mindfulness based stress reduction for healthy individuals: a meta-analysis. *J Psychosom Res.* 2015 Jun: 78(6): 519-528.

Chapter Eight:
Buscemi J, Kong A, Fitzgibbon M, et al. Society of Behavioral Medicine Position Statement: Elementary school-based physical activity supports academic achievement. *Transl Behav Med.* 2014 Dec; 4(4): 436-438.

Gapin JI, Laban JD, Etnier JL. The effects of physical activity on attention deficit hyperactivity disorder symptoms: the evidence. *Prev Med.* 2011 Jun; 52 Suppl 1: S70-74.

Vazou S, Smiley-Oyen A. Moving and academic learning are not antagonists: acute effects on executive function and enjoyment. *J Sport Exer Psychol.* 2014 Oct; 36(5): 474-485.

Chapter Nine:
Biswas A, Oh P, Faulkner G, et al. Sedentary time and its association with risk for disease incidence, mortality and hospitalization in adults: a systematic review and meta-analysis. *Ann Intern Med.* 2015; 162(2): 123-132.

Brito LB, Ricardo DR, Araujo DS, Ramos PS, Myers J, Araujo CG. Ability to sit and rise from the floor as a predictor of all-cause mortality. *Eur J Prev Cardiol.* 2014 Jul; 21(7): 892-898.

Chapter Ten:
Batista LH, Ferreira JJA, Rebelatto JR, Salvini TF. Active stretching improves flexibility, joint torque and functional mobility in older women. *Am J Phys Med Rehabil.* 2009 Oct; 88(10): 815-822.

Casperson CJ, Powell KE, Christenson GM. Physical activity, exercise, and physical fitness: definitions and distinctions for health-related research. *Public Health Rep.* 1985 March-April; 100(2): 126-129.

Klein S, Allison DB, Heymsfield SB, et al. Waist circumference and cardiometabolic risk: a consensus statement from Shaping America's Health: Association for Weight Management and Obesity Prevention; NAASO, The Obesity Society; the American Society for Nutrition; and the American Diabetes Association. *Obesity.* 2007 May; 15(5): 1061-1067.

Chapter Ten:
Lang T, Streeper T, Cawthon P, Baldwin K, Taaffe DR, Harris TB. Sarcopenia: etiology, clinical consequences, intervention, and assessment. *Osteoporos Int.* 2010; (21): 543-559.

Nelson ME, Rejeski WJ, Blair SN, et al. Physical activity and public health in older adults: Recommendations from the American College of Sports Medicine and the American Heart Association. *Circulation.* 2007; 116(9): 194-1105.

Newman AB, Kupelian V, Visser M, et al. Strength, but not muscle mass, is associated with mortality in the health, aging and body composition study cohort. *J Gerontol A Biol Sci Med Sci.* 2006; 61A(1): 72-77.

About the Author

Peggy Norwood Stella, M.A. knows the diet and fitness industry from the inside-out. After 30 years as an exercise professional promoting weight loss as the path to health, she now knows a better way and is offering her insights in her latest book: A New BMI - Why Body Mind Intelligence Matters More than Body Mass Index. She herself observed the struggles of many desperate "dieters" while serving as fitness director for the most prominent residential weight loss programs in the world, including Duke Diet and Fitness Center, Pritikin Longevity Center and Structure House.

When weight loss "success" started looking like an eating disorder and the majority of the "losers" regained, she started questioning her own role in perpetuating a diet mentality that seemed to do more harm than good. Realizing that there was far more to achieving health than focusing upon body weight, she created the concept of A New BMI.

Peggy's current mission is to educate, enlighten and inspire change from the current attitudes and beliefs about body and health, and to move towards a greater awareness of how the mind influences the body. Based upon her own observations and experiences working in the diet and fitness industry, she realizes the futility of focusing upon the scale as a measure of success. She knows the consequences of disconnecting from the body. She encourages two simple actions that make the greatest overall difference in creating health and well-being: Moving the body and quieting the mind.

Taking a mindful approach to moving the body helps the client engage with the body and enhances Body Mind Intelligence.

As an innovator in fitness education, she believes that a strong, positive relationship with the body will enhance quality of life and she encourages participation in activities such as dance, yoga and hiking in the woods. She is also certified in Equine Interactive Coaching and finds horses are the perfect teachers of connection with the body and with one's authentic self. Her company's name, Equessence LLC, reflects that connection.

As an exercise physiologist, movement educator and body advocate, Peggy encourages the practice of mindfulness combined with physical activity as the pathway to feeling better and moving better. She teaches her clients movement patterns that correct imbalances and improve overall posture, in addition to enhancing physical fitness. Her clients find that improving their movement patterns helps them enjoy greater mobility and vitality and therefore a higher quality of life overall.

Peggy embodies the physically active life. She has participated in the sport of gymnastics as both athlete and coach, and has won top honors as a competitive ballroom dancer in both American Rhythm and International Latin styles. She is a lifelong lover of horses and finds them to be the perfect teachers of connection with the body and with one's authentic self. Her workshops and retreats combine a wide variety of movement and restorative experiences, including forest meditations, yoga, dancing for the fun of it and learning self-awareness with horses.

She and her husband, Paul, enjoy daily hikes at the Eno River State Park, and the occasional tango lesson in their hometown of Durham, NC. She also enjoys riding and playing with her 10 year old Appaloosa named Dill.

Notes:

www.ingramcontent.com/pod-product-compliance
Lightning Source LLC
Chambersburg PA
CBHW052037270326

41931CB00012B/2531